Could
it be an
Allergy?

Could it be an Allergy?

Dr Joe Fitzgibbon

Newleaf

Newleaf

an imprint of
Gill & Macmillan Ltd
Goldenbridge
Dublin 8
with associated companies throughout the world
© Dr Joe Fitzgibbon 1998
0 7171 2682 X
Index compiled by Helen Litton
Design by O'K Graphic Design
Print origination by Andy Gilsenan
Printed by ColourBooks Ltd, Dublin

This book is typeset in 10/12 Garamond Book.

A catalogue record for this book is available from the British Library.

1 3 5 4 2

To Caoimhe, our latest arrival

Contents

Acknowledgments

I am indebted to those doctors who have gone before me as Clinical Allergists. They have, without exception, been gracious and willing teachers. Heartfelt thanks to Dr Sybil Birtwistle, Professor Jonathan Brostoff, Dr Keith Eaton, Dr Ronald Finn, Dr Alan Franklin, Dr Helen McEwen, Dr Jonathan Maberly, Dr John Mansfield, Dr Joe Miller, Dr Sarah Myhill and Dr Michael Radcliffe. Dr Len McEwen's unique contribution is acknowledged in chapter 18.

Although the following are probably not aware of their influence on my understanding of allergic disease, I would like to thank Professor Martin Church, Dr Steve Durham, Dr Alan Frankland, Dr Richard Pumphrey and Dr Veronica Varney.

My sincere thanks also to the many hospital specialists and family doctors who have supported and encouraged my work at the Allergy Clinic. A special word of thanks to Dr Deirdre Murphy for being particularly faithful in this regard.

Once again, I must thank Eveleen Coyle and her team at Gill & Macmillan for their skilled editorial advice. It goes without saying that this book would not exist without their invaluable help. Thanks also to Peter Lupson who inspired me to put pen to paper in the first place.

Finally, thanks to Aoife, who graciously carried more than her fair share while I was preoccupied with chapter and verse. She is a strong and faithful companion, and my greatest support.

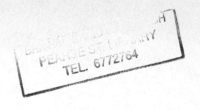

Introduction

An allergy is a hypersensitive reaction to an otherwise harmless substance in the environment. The allergic individual may thus react adversely to a wholesome food, a grass pollen or an animal dander. Indeed, the number of potential candidates here is endless, for it is possible to be allergic to anything under the sun — including the sun! The reactions themselves are equally diverse, ranging from simple itch to a potentially fatal collapse. Between these two extremes, there lies an excess of misery: the 'constant cold', sinus trouble, skin rash, and so the list goes on. Allergy, in the broadest sense of the word, is also said to play a part in many other ailments, such as hyperactivity, migraine, arthritis and chronic fatigue, to name but a few. Furthermore, allergic reactions may vary enormously from one patient to the next, and even within the same patient at different times. Thus, one person may sneeze in the presence of a horse, and another may wheeze. They are both allergic to the same thing, but they have very different reactions to it. Similarly, some allergies occur dramatically, within seconds of exposure to the offending agent; whereas others are more cumbersome, and take days or even weeks to develop. The former are usually well known to the patient, but the latter are seldom so.

Allergy is indeed a vast and fascinating field, replete with complexity and intrigue. This is, perhaps, the reason why it has become so entangled in controversy, and so muddled in the minds of doctor and patient alike. The greatest conflict arises between two schools of medical thought. The first relies heavily on objective tests, and maintains that 'If we cannot show the *mechanism* of an allergy (by skin-prick or blood test), then it's not an allergy.' The contrasting view is empirical, and much more comprehensive. It depends not on theory but on what we call clinical observation and experiment: 'If you get a symptom from an "otherwise harmless" substance, you are (to put it simply) allergic to it.' In this case, it does not matter whether we can understand the mechanism, it simply matters that we observe a symptom.

The strength of the first position is that it is built on 'hard science'. But herein also lies its weakness. As you can imagine, it is very reassuring to have a reliable test which gives objective evidence of allergy. It makes the job a lot easier! However, we cannot dismiss a suspected allergy on the basis of our present inability to 'prove it' in the laboratory. To do so would be to fall headlong into a scientific trap — a dark place where otherwise brilliant minds are restricted by the limitations of their machines. The purely scientific approach to allergy tests will lead to some patients being told that they are *not* allergic when, in fact, they *are*! Conversely, the broader proposition is founded on the art, rather than the science, of medicine. Once again, herein lie strength and weakness together. It is strong because it will consider greater possibilities. It will not dismiss what it cannot understand, and consequently will not easily 'miss' an allergy. It is weak because it cannot always prove the truth of its own diagnosis, and because it is prone to all the variables of human nature. In particular, it is vulnerable to the placebo effect: a mysterious, beguiling and often potent human response to the power of suggestion. In this case, some patients will be told that they *are* allergic when, in fact, they are *not*!

Although these opposing views are sometimes violently held, I believe that they both offer something to the allergic patient. In practice, it is possible to marry the warring factions. We can, with common sense, glean all that is good from each side of the argument and use it to our own advantage. By this means, I hope that you will develop a clear understanding of your own allergies. The great advantage of such knowledge is obvious: you can deal with the root cause of your symptoms, rather than suffer them or mindlessly suppress them with drugs. With this principle, we have a new and exciting avenue to explore in the search for permanent relief of hitherto intractable symptoms.

There is, however, one other source of confusion which must be addressed. I refer to the sheer bedlam generated in recent years by unqualified 'allergists'. These are self-appointed and unregulated practitioners who use very dubious 'tests' to tell unsuspecting patients what they are allergic to, usually a long list of foods. Many patients have followed prolonged and austere regimes on the basis of these 'results'. They will have done so with great expectation; and although some fortuitously improve, most obtain little or no benefit.

The fact that so many intelligent people adhere to these punishing diets is simply a measure of how desperate they are to rid themselves of symptoms. I admire them. They are proactive. They assume responsibility for their own health. They also display considerable determination in their search for a better quality of life, a life free from the constant harassment of sickness. Besides, their own doctors may not have been able to help, or may have failed to take them seriously when they enquired about allergy. Perhaps they were dismissed on the grounds of a negative blood test! This being so, they sought help where they thought they might find it. Desperation, however, is always a precarious state of mind. Diets 'prescribed' without medical or dietetic knowledge have resulted in many cases of nutritional deficiency. Tragically, there have also been a number of malnutrition-related deaths. How distressing it is when the innocent fall into the hands of the unscrupulous.

The essential question, then, is this: are *your* symptoms — whatever they may be — caused by a hypersensitive reaction to something 'otherwise harmless' in your environment; and if so, how can we pinpoint, exactly and reliably, what it is that causes you such grief? Finally, having identified your allergies, what can you do to secure a healthy and symptom-free future? The aim of this book is to provide you with clear answers to these very important questions. Indeed, you may discover that you have no allergies at all! In that case you will at least know that your answer lies elsewhere.

SECTION 1

What is an Allergy?

1   *The Range of Allergic Symptoms*

One of the difficulties facing us at the outset of any discussion on allergy is the sheer diversity of allergic symptoms. At first glance, the list of possible symptoms seems far too extensive to be credible. However, if you consider for a moment that virtually any organ in the body may be affected by an allergic reaction, you will begin to appreciate just why there are such manifold symptoms. And if you further consider that these reactions can be triggered by virtually anything in the environment, you cannot fail to be amazed at the enormousness of our task. Indeed, the work of an allergist is frequently compared to that of a detective. We must pick up allergic clues in the clinical history; we must sift through the environment at home, at work and at play, in our search for suspects; and we must apply a working knowledge of the underlying mechanisms of allergy, in so far as we understand them at the present time. Our difficulty is compounded by the fact that the symptoms of allergic disease may also occur in other diseases, and so we are duty-bound to ensure that there are no other explanations for the symptoms under investigation. Thus, rather than accepting allergic symptoms at face value, we must put them through the rigours of a thorough medical evaluation. Not all that sneezes, itches or wheezes is an allergy!

The vast majority of those who present themselves to an Allergy Clinic do so with one pressing question in mind. They want to know if their symptoms could be caused by allergy. This question leads to others: 'If there is a possibility that my symptoms are caused by allergy, how do I find out whether I have an allergy or not?' and 'If I do have an allergy, what on earth am I allergic to?' Doubtless, some of you already possess a fairly clear knowledge of what is causing your trouble. You would like to confirm your suspicions, and acquire a better understanding of your condition. You would also like, if feasible, to find an effective treatment. Others amongst you may feel confused. Perhaps you have been misled by questionable 'allergy tests', and are still pestered by symptoms in spite of your rigorous dieting. Most of you, however, will readily concede that you have no idea what you are allergic to, or even whether you have any allergies at all. You may have symptoms, of course, and symptoms with which you are only too familiar. You may also have a legacy of failed treatments, both orthodox and alternative, and you may still be searching for relief. Or you may simply feel uncomfortable about suppressing your symptoms with drugs, and you hope for a drug-free solution. You know instinctively that if you could discover the cause of your symptoms, you could also regain control of your health.

Most people are aware that the eyes, nose and lungs are frequently affected by allergic disease. The skin is also a well-recognised target for allergy. But other parts of the body are also likely to react, including the muscles and joints; the bladder and kidneys; the mouth and intestine; the heart and blood vessels; and even the brain itself. Remember, also, that allergy may occur in isolation, affecting just one part of the body; or as a multiple problem, affecting many organs at once. By way of illustration, allow me to construct a hypothetical 'day in the life' of an Allergy Clinic. Although this will of necessity be a limited view, it should help to impart a flavour of the myriad symptoms which may (or may not) have an allergic basis.

9 a.m. Peter

Our first patient is a four-year-old boy, whom we shall call Peter. (All names of patients have been changed.) He was referred by his family doctor with a number of problems. In the first place, his mother already knew that he was allergic to eggs. 'He breaks out in a rash if he so much as touches them!' she said. 'I gave him a spoonful once, when he was six months old, and he vomited for the whole day.' Sensibly, he was never given egg again. Peter, however, had other complaints. For instance, he had a cough that just wouldn't go away; and he wheezed when he became excited, or when he ran about. These are the symptoms of asthma. He also had a 'runny' nose, which he was in the habit of rubbing in a very typical way. He would press the tip of his nose onto the pad of his middle finger and run his

4

hand skywards with a big sniff. We call it the 'allergic salute', and he had a permanent horizontal crease on his nose to show for it. In addition, he had dry, itchy skin. He was always scratching himself, and in his sleep would frequently draw blood by tearing at the worst-affected sites. We call this eczema. Finally, and as if that wasn't enough to contend with, he was hyperactive. Peter's mother noticed particularly bad behaviour whenever he ate certain foods. Oranges and biscuits, for example, would 'send him wild'. Cutting these out of his diet helped a little, but did not solve the problem. His parents wondered whether some other food, still in his diet, was affecting his conduct.

Skin tests revealed that Peter was very sensitive to house dust mites. This allergy may well be relevant to many of his symptoms, including his asthma, nasal allergy and eczema. We also went through a standard assessment for hyperactivity. His score on the rating scale was indeed suggestive of a problem in this area. Moreover, there were good reasons to suspect that food was a contributing factor in his case: he already had a known sensitivity to egg, his behaviour was noticeably worse after eating certain foods, and he had all of the other allergic conditions mentioned above. There is, however, no reliable skin or blood test to help us with his hyperactivity. A formal and painstaking investigation of his diet is the only way to determine which foods, if any, are contributing to his difficult behaviour.

9.30 a.m. Mark

Our next patient, Mark, is a 35-year-old farmer who has returned to the Allergy Clinic for review. When he first attended some months ago he complained of 'sinus and chest trouble'. His nose was constantly 'bunged up'. Sometimes it poured like a tap, especially when he got one of those sneezing attacks. It used to take him an age to fall asleep at night because he could not breathe properly. He woke in the mornings 'with a throat like sandpaper', dry and sore — a common complaint in those who (for whatever reason) breathe through their mouth during sleep. He also had a wheeze for as long as he could remember, but this had become much worse in recent years, and his inhalers were not as effective as they once were. What worried him most, however, was the fact that his livelihood was now at stake. 'When I visit the market all of my old symptoms flare up, and I get new ones too,' he explained. His eyes would become red and 'itch like crazy' within minutes of contact with cattle.

Doing business under these circumstances had become increasingly difficult for him. After investigation, Mark was found to be allergic to dust mites and cattle. He also had some degree of food allergy. He responded very nicely to treatment, and was now able to breathe easily, sleep through the night, and attend the mart with minimal symptoms.

10 a.m. Karen

Karen is a ten-year-old girl who has returned with her parents for the results of a blood test. A few weeks earlier, she had experienced a rather frightening swelling of her mouth together with an intense itch of the tongue after eating fish. Her father pointed out that she had since developed similar symptoms after using a fork which had previously been used on fish. And yet, in spite of such a clear and dramatic clinical history, the blood test came back negative. We were, therefore, still no wiser, and it was now time to proceed to skin tests. By way of precaution, and because we did not want to spark off an allergic attack in such a sensitive patient, we diluted the fish extract 15,000 times! Within ten minutes Karen had produced a skin reaction to even this tiny amount, confirming that she was indeed extremely sensitive to fish. The rest of this visit was spent in conversation with Karen and her parents. We covered several important topics. She must now avoid fish in any guise and at all costs. The next allergic reaction could be much more serious; in fact, this is a potentially life-threatening allergy. She needed instruction on self-treatment in an emergency, and needed to understand that these precautions could never be relaxed. They must become a way of life for her, and remain so for the rest of her days.

11 a.m. Joyce

Joyce has done really well. She had been dogged by ill health for the best part of fifteen years. She had frequent migraine headaches; joint and muscle pains; digestive problems (indigestion, abdominal discomfort and bloating, and bouts of diarrhoea); asthma; chronic sinus trouble; and debilitating fatigue. Actually, she was so tired that she often fell asleep at her desk in the office! Although hopeful, Joyce thought it unlikely that she was allergic to foods. 'It couldn't be a food, doctor, because I'm not eating anything new.' This is a common misunderstanding. It is only ever possible to become allergic to something if we have come across it before, in some form or other. To prove the point, Joyce had lost all of her symptoms within ten days of adopting a prescribed diet. Her head was clear, her joints were free, her tummy was quiet and she could smell again. She could not remember when she had last felt so well. As she expanded her diet she reacted adversely to many foods, including onion, mushroom, melon, wheat, dairy produce, corn and malt. Today we discussed an effective treatment which would, in time, enable Joyce to eat these foods without getting symptoms.

11.30 a.m. Mary

Mary has also come back for review. She is a twenty-year-old student who was plagued with recurrent swellings of the eyes and lips. So disfiguring were these swellings that she was too embarrassed to leave her lodgings. She also told me about an itchy rash which covered her whole body, and a long-standing history of asthma. She noticed that her asthma was much worse when the rash flared, and that she had a 'constant cold'. She then told me a very interesting fact: all symptoms got worse when she took an aspirin for headache. This was an important clue. Although Mary was not aware of it, some 25 per cent of her regularly eaten foods contain a substance very similar (but not identical) to aspirin. Furthermore, this 'triad' of itchy rash, asthma and nasal problems is sometimes associated with aspirin sensitivity. She had now completed one month on a 'low-aspirin' diet. 'It's great!' she said, 'I have had no swelling or itch, and I have missed no lectures as a result.' 'But what about the asthma and nasal symptoms?' I enquired eagerly. 'Oh, they're as bad as ever,' she said. Back to the drawing board! Aspirin-containing foods were obviously relevant to some of her symptoms, but not to others. Skin tests revealed a sensitivity to grass pollen and dust mites. Given that it was the wrong time of year for grass pollen symptoms, we now concentrated on dust mites, and the various measures Mary could adopt to reduce her exposure to these.

12 a.m. Sandra

Sandra has come to the Allergy Clinic today because she is convinced that certain foods are making her ill. She gives a very long and complex history, characterised mostly by symptoms of depression. Some years ago she was admitted to a psychiatric hospital, and she enjoyed considerable benefit from treatment at the time. The diagnosis of depression, however, did not sit comfortably with her then, and still unsettles her today. She is now tired. Her memory and concentration are impaired, her sleep is restless and unrefreshing, and she feels short of breath. She also complains of frequent headache, poor appetite and muscle pains. After a while, Sandra admitted rather reluctantly that her marriage was on the rocks, and had been for some time. Moreover, things had come to a head recently, and there was talk of separation. In the recent past, she brought herself to an 'allergist'. There she was told that her problems were caused by food allergy. She had since avoided a number of foods in the firm belief that she was 'allergic' rather than 'depressed'. Her symptoms, however, did not improve, and hence her visit to the clinic today. She was quite sure that some other food, as yet unidentified, was holding her down.

Having listened carefully to her sad story, I had several reasons to doubt the 'allergic' theory, and I expressed my doubts to Sandra. We now found ourselves in a conflict of attribution: the patient attributes her symptoms to one thing, whilst her doctor attributes them to another. This is a crucial moment for Sandra. If she vigorously defends her 'not depressed' position when she is in fact depressed, she will not get the help she so badly needs, and will remain depressed. If on the other hand I am wrong, she will suffer the same fate. The only way to resolve this question is to invite Sandra to challenge her own belief. She can do this by agreeing to a supervised investigation of her diet. The first step is to eat all omitted foods for a period of two weeks. If this brings about a significant worsening of symptoms, she may be on the right track after all. If she is right, she should then notice a dramatic and lasting improvement on a prescribed Low Allergy Diet. From my experience with other patients in the same boat, I expect Sandra to return in a fortnight with no appreciable change in her symptoms. My hope is that she will then be ready to explore the deeper psychosocial factors which trouble her so.

12.30 p.m. Margaret

Margaret first presented seven months ago with a two-year history of a very itchy rash. She was only eleven years old at the time, but had already noticed that her rash was much worse if she ate anything with artificial colours or preservatives. Her observation was confirmed by the complete disappearance of rash on a prescribed diet which was free of these substances.

Since then, she has had four injections to switch off (desensitise) her allergy. Last month I sent her away with instructions to test herself with a well-known brand of confectionery, one made up almost entirely of chemicals! I was pleased to hear that she could now eat all foods without problem. It's not that I would encourage her to gorge on 'junk food', but I did want her to enjoy a greater freedom of choice.

2 p.m. Michael

Michael is a 42-year-old horticulturist who has turned to lettuce in recent years for a living. He has several growing tunnels which produce a fine crop. Recently, however, he developed a rash on both hands. This was aggravated by handling the plant at harvest time. He was quite sure that lettuce was not his problem because he has been handling it for some years now, and besides, he is able to handle the young plant with impunity. He suspects that a mould, which lives on lettuce, is causing his trouble. After further enquiry, it transpires that Michael also starts to wheeze in the tunnels, particularly when the crop is being loaded for transport to the market. As with Joyce, seen earlier in the day, Michael did not know that he could become allergic to something 'out of the blue', so to speak. The truth is, the more often we have contact with a substance, the more likely we are to become allergic to it! This explains why surgeons and nurses become allergic to their gloves, why bakers become allergic to flour, why painters become allergic to paint, and so on. Furthermore, Michael was also unaware that the adult lettuce leaf contains a substance which the young leaf does not yet possess, and that this is the substance to which he has developed an allergy.

Skin tests confirmed his sensitivity to the adult leaf, and ruled out an allergy to the mould. He must now seriously consider his future. If he stays on, his wheeze is likely to develop into full-blown asthma, and if he persists further, he could remain asthmatic even after he abandons lettuce for a different crop.

2.30 p.m. Anne

Anne is a 35-year-old mother of two who works in the textile industry. She presented with a number of baffling complaints. First and foremost, she is quite depressed, and does not hesitate to say so. Furthermore, she has a fairly good idea what makes her feel so low. There is no doubt, however, that she also suffers from allergy. Last year, for example, she broke out in a rash after a visit to the hairdresser. Her scalp and neck were affected at first, but then the rash spread to her upper chest and back. Quite nasty it was too, but at least she could understand it, and it seemed to settle down after a while. What baffled her now, however, was the similar rash which recurred in spite of her staying away from hair colours. Her doctor tried to help by ordering a blood test for allergy, and this threw up some interesting results. She was, on blood test, allergic to wheat, egg, milk, soy and peanut! Anne therefore stayed away from these foods as best she could, but she still ate them from time to time in small quantities. Were these small amounts, she wondered, still causing her trouble?

Skin tests confirmed her allergy to hair dye. They also revealed an allergy to nickel. Significantly, the dye is also found in leathers, and nickel is present in fasteners and zips. Anne is in regular contact with these substances at work. Many of her symptoms disappeared away from work and on a prescribed diet. The subsequent (closely supervised) food reintroductions were largely uneventful. In other words, although her blood test suggested that many food allergies were present, these were not at all relevant to her symptoms. These are referred to as dormant, or latent, allergies, and they may remain dormant for a lifetime. This example brings home the wise words of an esteemed elderly colleague: 'Allergy tests should not be relied upon to tell us what we don't know, they should be used only to confirm our clinical suspicions.' What Anne did discover, however, was that an accumulation of artificial chemicals in food, together with the other chemicals referred to above, were the combined cause of her skin trouble. She felt considerably lighter in mood once her problem was sorted out.

3 p.m. Mrs Talbot

Mrs Talbot is a 65-year-old woman who has arthritis in her hips. One of these is now so painful that she has decided to go ahead with a hip replacement. She told the orthopaedic surgeon about her allergy to jewellery, and about a rash she had on both sides of her face. The pattern of this rash was very suggestive of an allergy to her spectacle frames. These are the typical symptoms of nickel allergy. The surgeon requested a full evaluation of Mrs Talbot's allergies before proceeding with the operation. He knew, of course, that most hip replacements contain nickel, and that the new (metal) hip would not last long if she was allergic to it. Skin tests had been applied forty-eight hours previously and it was now time to read the results. As expected, Mrs Talbot had a very strongly positive reaction to nickel. She had an equally strong reaction to cobalt, another metal. These metals frequently cross-react, i.e. if you are allergic to one, you are very likely to be allergic to the other. What we did not expect, however, was the strong reaction to rubber and certain disinfectants. We were now in a position to advise the surgeon that his suspicions were correct, and that he should use a cobalt- and nickel-free hip. He was further able to prevent a potentially nasty allergic reaction during the operation itself by avoiding the use of rubber gloves and the aforementioned disinfectant.

3.30 p.m. David

David looks better! When I first saw him four weeks ago he was in an awful state. He is a 41-year-old business executive who presented with a twenty-five-year history of 'embarrassing itch'. He described a burning painful itch on his bottom and in 'the back passage'. Over the years he had tried every sort of cream and potion imaginable, but without joy. Whatever self-control he had during waking hours was lost during sleep. He frequently woke in the night to find himself tearing at the itch, but the more he scratched, the worse it got. This incessant interruption of his sleep had finally left him exhausted, and was very likely the reason behind his muscular aches and pains, and his feeling of general malaise. David confirmed that he felt marvellous — in fact, he couldn't get over it himself. All he had done between his first visit and today's review was adopt a different form of toilet hygiene. It was not a question of improving his cleanliness, for he was perfectly clean; we just wanted to give him a rest from toilet tissue! 'I didn't tell you last time, doctor, because I thought it would sound crazy, but whenever the itch was at its worst, I used to sneeze a lot! Now, my itch has completely cleared up, and my nose is no longer blocked!' Consequently, he was able to enjoy refreshing sleep for the first time in ages, his exhaustion was gone and he no longer had aching muscles.

David is allergic to formaldehyde, a well-known source of allergic symptoms. Toilet tissue, and other tissue papers, are impregnated with this substance during manufacture. Whenever toilet tissue containing formaldehyde was brought into contact with his skin, it sparked off the allergic itch. Simply handling tissue would be enough to spark off his allergic nose. Think about that for a moment! You get a bit of a sniffle so you reach for a tissue. Then you have an allergic reaction to the tissue. But you think this is just a bit more of the original sniffle so you reach for another tissue. Before you know where you are, you have a permanent allergic nose caused by the very tissues you use to blow your nose!

4 p.m. Paula

Paula is now towards the end of her dietary investigation for food allergy. She has suffered from rheumatoid arthritis for the past thirty years. Ever since her fifteenth birthday she has been on a roller-coaster ride of joint stiffness, pain and swelling. Over the past year, however, her symptoms had become more persistent. In addition, she complained of fluid retention (swollen ankles and bloated abdomen), sinus problems and fatigue. Before she embarked on this diet, she had morning stiffness in most joints for about thirty minutes. Thereafter, she would feel a bit better, but sitting down for any length of time would quickly lead to her joints 'seizing up' again. Within fourteen days of a prescribed diet she reported that she was no longer stiff in the mornings, she had much less pain, and she had taken no arthritis tablets for the previous five days — a feat heretofore unimaginable for her. Her symptom diary showed clear reactions to chicken, cabbage, soy, yeast and wheat, with minor reactions to banana and beef. Between reactions she remained perfectly well. If she wanted to, she could now continue to expand her diet, find as many safe foods as possible, and simply avoid the offending foods. However, Paula wants to try a course of desensitisation because she leads far too busy a life to be forever watching her diet.

4.30 p.m. Marie

Marie suspects that she has 'candida', and that she is allergic to yeast. She has been troubled by many symptoms over the years, such as bloating of the abdomen, constipation, fatigue and headaches. She finds it hard to get off to sleep, and her mood swings have become more pronounced, causing much personal and family unhappiness. Marie also told me about a family tragedy which took place shortly before she became ill. Some time after this she read a book about 'candida' in which she found many of her symptoms explained, as she thought, and she has been dieting ever since. She has spent a small fortune on doctors and unqualified practitioners. Marie's symptoms only partially responded to diet, but this had not weakened her resolve. I was alarmed at her weight, a mere six and a half stone when it should have been nine! I was also concerned that her menstrual periods were scanty, and that her present diet was grossly deficient in calcium. I took a blood test three weeks ago to find out if she did have a problem with yeast overgrowth in the bowel. Then I asked her to go home and eat everything she could lay her hands on, including the foods she had been so strenuously avoiding. I was afraid that she had an eating disorder, such as anorexia nervosa, and was using the 'candida' as a cover-up; or that she was trying as best she could to hide the fact that she had lost her appetite in the aftermath of the family tragedy, a tragedy from which she had not yet recovered.

The results of her blood test are available to us today. They confirm the presence of a very small overgrowth of yeast, but this is not, in any way, sufficient to explain her symptoms. Meanwhile, Marie has enjoyed eating all manner of foods over the past few weeks, and has managed to put on a little weight. A short course of anti-yeast medication, without dietary restriction, will quickly restore balance to the bowel. I will invite her to return in one month to review her progress. Whatever symptoms remain at that stage cannot be attributed to 'candida', but may well respond to other, perhaps more appropriate, forms of treatment.

5 p.m.

The end of what you might call an absorbing day! But as you can appreciate, it is impossible to represent the full scope of allergic symptoms within the context of a single day in the clinic. Indeed, I could fill this book with case histories as fascinating as these, and still have more to tell. However, we need to move on now, and spend a little time looking at the immune system. In so doing, you will begin to understand the mechanisms by which allergic symptoms develop. Before we leave the subject of symptoms, have a look at the following drawing, which summarises the possible manifestations of allergic disease.

Possible symptoms of allergy

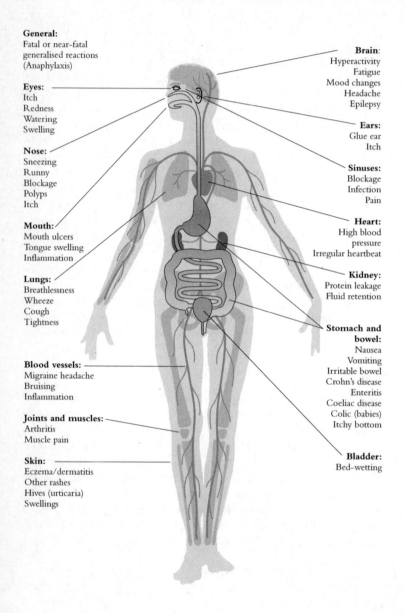

General:
Fatal or near-fatal
generalised reactions
(Anaphylaxis)

Eyes:
Itch
Redness
Watering
Swelling

Nose:
Sneezing
Runny
Blockage
Polyps
Itch

Mouth:
Mouth ulcers
Tongue swelling
Inflammation

Lungs:
Breathlessness
Wheeze
Cough
Tightness

Blood vessels:
Migraine headache
Bruising
Inflammation

Joints and muscles:
Arthritis
Muscle pain

Skin:
Eczema/dermatitis
Other rashes
Hives (urticaria)
Swellings

Brain:
Hyperactivity
Fatigue
Mood changes
Headache
Epilepsy

Ears:
Glue ear
Itch

Sinuses:
Blockage
Infection
Pain

Heart:
High blood
pressure
Irregular heartbeat

Kidney:
Protein leakage
Fluid retention

**Stomach and
bowel:**
Nausea
Vomiting
Irritable bowel
Crohn's disease
Enteritis
Coeliac disease
Colic (babies)
Itchy bottom

Bladder:
Bed-wetting

2 The Range of Allergic Reactions

I have no wish to write a lengthy or complicated essay on the delicate wonders of the immune system, and I am sure that you have no desire to read one! But I would like to offer a very brief introduction to the subject. This should help us to understand the context and mechanisms of allergy.

The role of the immune system in health

Protection from infection

The immune system has several very important functions to perform. In the first place, the immune system is remarkable for its ability to defend us from the numerous threats we face in our environment. It has the ability to recognise what belongs to itself, and to distinguish 'self' from everything else it encounters ('non-self'). The system is on constant patrol, always alert to the possibility of invasion. Thus, when a microscopic bug, such as a virus, tries to infect the body, the immune system quickly identifies the bug as 'foreign' and sounds the alarm. The battle which follows gives rise to the symptoms of inflammation. Tonsillitis, for example, is an inflammation (immune reaction or battle) in the tonsils as they deal with infection. Once the battle is over, the system commits a specific line of defence to memory, thus ensuring a more prompt and efficient handling of the next attempted invasion by that particular organism. This is the principle behind immunity to infection and immunisation (vaccination).

Protection from cancer

Secondly, there are times when the threat of invasion comes from within the body itself, in the form of cancer. Cancerous cells arise from previously healthy cells as they divide and replicate. If the replication goes wrong, the cell may assume a life of its own and may then ignore the normal rules of growth and fair play. These rogue cells now pose a threat, because if they are not stopped quickly they will give rise to malignancy. Thankfully, the immune system has a 'military police' facility which recognises these harmful cells, brands them as non-self, and targets them for destruction before they cause disease.

How does the immune system work?

The first step of immune defence is **recognition.** The special cells that **recognise** the difference between self and non-self are called lymphocytes. They live mostly in the lymph glands and bloodstream — where there are some sixteen billion of them in circulation at any one time! Each one keeps its eyes peeled, so to speak, and raises the alarm when suspicious foreign materials or unhealthy cancerous cells are encountered. The second great skill of immune defence is the ability to **respond** efficiently once an alarm is raised. The immune **response** involves several different cell types, each with its own job to do, together with a host of specialist proteins. Some of these proteins are aligned in cascades, somewhat like a row of dominoes: once the whistle blows and the first domino falls, the whole series will follow suit. Each protein in the cascade sparks off activity in the next until the last protein overcomes the invader with a lethal thrust. Complete annihilation of the enemy is achieved by the immune-equivalent of a garbage disposal system: immune cells literally engulf and consume the wounded foreign material.

Antibodies also play a vital role in our protection, in terms of both their ability to recognise foreign matter and their readiness to join in the assault on it. They are highly specialised proteins known also as **immunoglobulins**, and are divided into five main categories: A, D, E, G and M. We will be particularly interested in immunoglobulin E (IgE), a highly reactive antibody, responsible for many of the symptoms of allergy.

What can go wrong with the immune system?

The immune system is prone to failure in several realms.
  It may . . .

- fail to mount an effective challenge to infection
- fail to keep the lid on malignant change, giving rise to cancer
- fail to discern between self and non-self, causing autoimmune disease
- overreact to a harmless substance, causing allergy

Infection

Some bugs are able to escape the effective attention of our immune systems, even in relative health. These will cause disease. Examples include the bacillus which causes tuberculosis, and the parasite which causes malaria, but there are many others too numerous to mention here. However, unless we have healthy immune systems, we will succumb to recurrent and sometimes overwhelming infection by bugs which we should have been able to handle with comparative ease. Thus, if we are unable to produce sufficient quantities of antibody, immune protein or lymphocytes, we will end up in a state of immune deficiency. This is one of the main problems faced by patients with AIDS (Acquired Immune Deficiency Syndrome): they are unable to defend themselves against foreign invasion because their lymphocytes are infected and killed by the human immunodeficiency virus (HIV).

Cancer

The potentially malignant events mentioned above occur regularly in us all, and our immune systems are usually very good at mopping them up. Thus, cancer, when it does occur, is a failure of the normal immune surveillance mechanism.

Autoimmune disease

Sometimes the immune system fails to discern between self and non-self. It may initiate an attack against the body's own healthy cells. The inflammatory (immune) response that ensues is auto-destructive: the body is destroying a part of its own healthy self. Staying with the analogy of war, this is the tragedy of so-called friendly fire. The resulting diseases are referred to as auto-immune diseases. Examples include some forms of arthritis and kidney disease.

Allergy

Finally, the immune system may overreact to a harmless substance in the mistaken belief that it poses a threat to health. This is what happens in allergy. To put it another way, an allergy is an overkill, in which the immune system bears down heavily on some quite innocent substance from the environment. The substance will not cause suffering or pain, and it will not invade the body like an infectious organism. It is, by its very nature, truly harmless. The allergic reaction, on the other hand, by its violence, causes a great deal of misery and, sadly, may even cause death. Any substance capable of inciting an allergic reaction is called an **allergen**. Thus, we speak of the dust mite allergen, pollen and mould allergens, peanut allergen, and so forth. In clinical practice, most allergic patients will react to several allergens, some will react to just one or two, and a few hapless patients will react to many.

More about allergy

The word 'allergy' was coined in 1906 by a Viennese paediatrician, Clemens von Pirquet. He used it to describe the violent reactions which some of his young patients had to vaccination injections. These patients, he said, had an abnormal response to the serum commonly used in the vaccines of his day. They were in a state of what he called 'altered reactivity' (Greek *állos érgon*) — they had allergy. Although medical practitioners quickly recognised these states of altered reactivity in their own patients, they were quite baffled by them. So it was, in the 1920s, that they referred to allergic disease as 'atopy', which, literally translated, means 'a strange disease'! Atopy is still used in clinical practice today in reference to allergic individuals and their families; and sometimes to describe specific diseases, such as atopic dermatitis (eczema).

The discovery of IgE

Our understanding of these allergies was greatly enhanced by the discovery, in 1967, of the highly reactive antibody alluded to above, namely IgE. In health, IgE protects us from invasion by intestinal parasites. It has the ability to recognise them, and to initiate an appropriate immune response to them. Unfortunately, in susceptible individuals, it also recognises harmless foreign material, such as pollen, animal dander, food, and so on. In other words, these patients are hypersensitive: their IgE pays a great deal of attention to things it should ignore. The resulting immune response is inappropriate, and this is what gives rise to the symptoms of allergy. Furthermore, allergic patients frequently produce an excessive amount of IgE, which compounds their problem.

With the discovery of IgE came the exciting prospect of a simple diagnostic test for allergy. Doctors could now measure the total amount of IgE in a patient's blood (to see if it was high), and determine specifically what allergens their IgE was recognising and reacting to. Furthermore, researchers started to unravel the mysteries of how IgE reacts with allergen, so much so that we now understand a great deal about the entire mechanism. However, our excitement was curtailed by the fact that some individuals develop allergic symptoms without the involvement of IgE. The converse was also found: some people have IgE which recognises things that they are not yet allergic to (but they may become so with time). So, although it is clear that IgE is a major player in allergic disease, it is equally clear that there is much more to the story.

Different types of allergy

Some understanding of these non-IgE allergies came from the realisation that other antibodies could also react adversely with harmless allergens, albeit in very different ways. For the sake of convenience, we now classify these different hypersensitive reactions into four distinct types. We are aware, in so doing, that such distinctions are somewhat artificial, especially when we leave the laboratory and face a patient. Nevertheless, they do help us to appreciate the variety of allergic mechanisms which occur in the immune system. The four types of hypersensitivity are briefly summarised.

Type 1 hypersensitivity is one which occurs immediately or very soon after contact with an allergen. These are usually IgE-driven. Type 1 allergies are associated with chest (asthma), skin (dermatitis and urticaria), nasal (hay fever and sinus trouble) and eye (conjunctivitis) allergies. They are also responsible for most fatal and near-fatal reactions (anaphylaxis).

Type 2 hypersensitivity reactions are driven by IgG and IgM antibodies. These bind directly to cell walls and lead to their destruction. In health, this reaction protects us from invading parasites and so on. The antibodies bind to the parasite (which is, after all, nothing more than a cell) and prepare it for destruction by other components of the immune system. But when the antibodies bind to cells in a blood transfusion or in a donated kidney graft, they wreck havoc — causing blood transfusion reactions and graft rejections. Finally, if they bind to our own tissues, they produce autoimmune disease, such as nephritis (inflammation of the kidneys).

Type 3 hypersensitivity reactions are also driven by IgG and IgM antibodies. In this case, however, they bind not to cell walls, but to allergen floating free in the bloodstream. When allergen is bound to antibody in this way, it forms an 'immune complex' — a microscopic clump of immune garbage. These are normally mopped up by 'garbage disposal cells' in the immune system; but if they are too numerous, or if the immune system cannot handle them for any other reason, they are dumped into other tissues, causing a great deal of damage. This is what happens in rheumatoid arthritis, and in some forms of allergy involving mould, vegetable, paint and wood.

Type 4 hypersensitivity reactions are unique. They are *delayed reactions* in which immune cells (not antibodies) react against an allergen *over time*. This is the underlying mechanism of contact allergy in the skin.

For practical purposes I have divided the book into several sections. You have just finished section 1. In section 2 we will consider the most common allergic problems; and in section 3 we will take a look at fatal and near-fatal allergy. Both of these sections deal mainly with the hypersensitivity reactions described above. Then, in sections 4 and 5, we will deal with other types of allergy (states of altered reactivity) that are not, as yet, so easily measured or understood. We will also examine the vexed questions of 'candida' and chemical sensitivity, and pay tribute to the importance of mind–body–mind interactions. Finally, in section 6, we will look at reliable allergy tests and effective allergy treatment.

SECTION 2

Common Allergic Problems

3.1 Allergy and the Skin: Eczema

Healthy skin

Although it may not appear immediately obvious, the skin is a very important organ. Indeed, it is the largest organ in the body, and it has several vital functions to perform.

The skin . . .

- affords a layer of protection from noxious substances in the environment
- is water-resistant and protects us from leaking our own fluids!
- plays an important role in temperature regulation
- helps to rid the body of toxins and waste products by sweating them out
- allows us to feel the difference between hot and cold, rough and smooth, pain and pleasure, etc.
- Finally — and this may come as a surprise — the skin is an integral part of the immune system. It contains many cells which belong to the immune system, and we shall meet these in due course as we look at how allergies affect the skin.

CASE HISTORY

Ten-year-old Dermot was referred to the Allergy Clinic because he had an intensely itchy rash. It first appeared in infancy, when he was just four months old. At the time only his face was affected, and he was successfully treated with medicated creams prescribed by his doctor. As he got older the rash reappeared, and spread to other parts of his body, including his neck, arms, legs and ankles. The rest of his skin, although not directly affected by rash, was dry and flaky. In recent months his rash had worsened considerably, and his ferocious scratching had left him with large areas of broken and weeping skin. He was in pain. He was also miserable because the itch had disrupted his sleep for weeks, and because his peers at school were now teasing him about his appearance. Dermot has **eczema**.

What is eczema?

Eczema is a term rather loosely applied to a wide range of chronic inflammatory skin conditions. It derives from a Greek word meaning to 'boil out' or 'ooze'. There are numerous different kinds of eczema, but the commonest by far is atopic eczema, also known as atopic dermatitis. In practice, we refer to it simply as eczema. The characteristic feature of eczema is a dry, inflamed skin. The sequence of events is easy to understand: dry, inflamed skin is itchy, itchy skin is scratched, scratched skin breaks down and weeps, and broken skin may become infected. As broken skin heals, it goes through an itchy phase, and this sparks off more scratching. Chronic scratching and rubbing ultimately lead to thickening of the skin. Thickened skin assumes a red or silvery sheen which we call lichenification. Other colour changes may also occur involving the accumulation or loss of pigment. This will show up as patches of 'tanned' skin on a pale background (hyperpigmentation), or as pale patches on a dark background (hypopigmentation).

Who gets it?

Eczema is an increasingly common disease of early infancy and childhood. Indeed, it has become so common since the Second World War that we can now expect some 20 per cent of all children to be affected at some stage in their youth. Of these, 60 per cent will develop the condition during their first year of life. Most of the others will get it before they reach their fifth birthday.

Will they grow out of it?

It is often said that children grow out of their eczema. This is a true statement, but it needs some qualification. Two-thirds of infants (less than one year old) with eczema will be free of symptoms by the age of five; and half of the children who develop eczema after their first birthday will be trouble-free by the time they reach their mid-teens. In the most encouraging studies, up to 90 per cent become symptom-free in their adult lives. However, almost all patients will 'carry' their dry skin into adulthood. This will predispose them to occasional attacks of eczema. They may also find themselves prone to irritant dermatitis (see chapter 3.II). Some individuals will retain their eczema throughout life.

What causes it?

We do not know the cause of eczema, but we do know that there is a genetic factor involved. For example, if one identical twin has eczema, the other twin has an 86 per cent chance of getting it as well. In other words, the tendency towards eczema is passed on in the genes. We also know that eczema is frequently complicated by allergic and non-allergic triggers. However, it is not correct to assume that allergy is involved in each and every case of eczema. We are faced therefore with a two-edged responsibility. We must identify those eczematous individuals in whom allergy is important, and distinguish them from those in whom it is not. The former will benefit by the knowledge that they *are allergic*: for they can now avoid and/or treat their allergies. The latter will benefit by the knowledge that they are *not allergic*: for they can now rest assured that they are not aggravating their condition by what they eat or touch. In eczema there are three main allergic triggers which are worthy of consideration:

1. allergy to the foods we eat
2. allergy to things in the air we breathe (house dust mites and pollen)
3. allergy to the things we touch (contact allergy)

1. Food allergy and eczema

There is no doubt that food allergy plays a role in many cases of eczema. Some researchers suggest that as many as 70 per cent of children with eczema will improve on appropriate diets. Others suggest that the true figure is closer to 30 per cent. In any case, it is clear that the role of food allergy should be considered, particularly if the patient is not responding to other forms of treatment. The diagnosis of food allergy in eczema may be suggested by skin and blood tests. However, the best test of all is the Low Allergy Diet. Briefly stated, the Low Allergy Diet consists of ten to twelve foods rarely eaten by the patient heretofore. The patient eats as much as they like of these foods for a period of ten days. Patients with food allergy will notice a dramatic reduction in itch whilst on the diet, and an equally dramatic recurrence of itch when allergic trigger foods are reintroduced to the diet. (See chapter 17 for a full description of the Low Allergy Diet.)

2. House dust mites, pollen and eczema

House dust mites do not cause eczema, but they can certainly make it worse. This is true if — and only if — the eczematous patient is allergic to them. This is how it works. You will recall that eczematous skin is dry and inflamed, that dry skin is itchy, that itchy skin is scratched, and that scratched skin breaks down. Once the skin surface is broken in this way, the dust mite allergen (the bit that causes the allergy) gets into the skin. The allergen is now in direct contact with the immune system, and it sparks off an allergic reaction. The role of dust mite allergy in eczema, then, is very much a secondary event. The primary event is the breakdown of skin, the body's natural defensive barrier. The secondary event, in those allergic to the house dust mite, is the allergic reaction now raging in the already inflamed skin.

An identical situation arises when grass or other pollen enters the broken eczematous skin of pollen-sensitive individuals. These secondary allergic phenomena greatly complicate the healing process. It stands to reason, therefore, that those who are allergic to these allergens should adopt measures to reduce their exposure to them. They will be rewarded by a significant reduction in symptoms. It is equally obvious that allergen avoidance measures are a waste of time and effort for those who are not allergic to them. For full details on house dust mite avoidance measures see appendix 1.

How do I find out if I am allergic to house dust mites or pollen?

The diagnosis of dust mite and pollen allergy is very straightforward. A small drop of allergen is placed on the forearm, and the underlying skin is pricked with a tiny pin. An itchy hive will develop at the site of the pinprick within fifteen minutes in allergic individuals. The larger the hive, the more sensitive the patient, and the more relevant the allergy to that individual. There will be no hive in patients who are not allergic to the allergens. Diagnosis may also be secured by a blood test called the RAST, although skin tests are faster, more extensive and probably more reliable (see chapter 17).

3. Contact allergy and eczema

Some people develop an allergic rash from simply touching (or 'contacting') things they are allergic to. There are two forms of contact allergy: those which occur within seconds or minutes of contact, and those which develop very slowly over days or weeks. These two forms of allergy are quite readily distinguished from each other by their appearance. The former consists of hives and is referred to as contact urticaria (see chapter 3.III). The latter, known as contact allergic dermatitis, assumes an appearance identical to the rash of eczema. This is what makes it so important to patients with eczema. How can they be sure that their eczema is not in fact a contact allergic dermatitis? They certainly cannot tell by simply looking at the rash, and nor can their doctor always tell. Furthermore, the rash of contact dermatitis may spread quite a distance from the site of contact. Thus, nickel allergy (which affects 5 to 10 per cent of women) may spread from the skin under a nickel-containing watch strap to affect the entire length of the arm. It is easy to imagine how such a patient can quickly develop a widespread and apparently random rash from contact with other nickel-containing items such as zips, buckles, buttons, studs, keys, coins, and the like. Very rarely, eczema may be driven by an obscure contact allergy, such as an allergy to the mercury in your dental fillings. The diagnosis of contact dermatitis must be confirmed or excluded by patch tests. This involves strapping a number of suspect allergens on the skin of the back, and leaving them in place for forty-eight hours. Allergic reactions are then read by the allergist. (For more details on patch tests see chapter 17.)

The non-allergic triggers of eczema include:

1. false food allergy
2. contact with irritant substances (see chapter 3.II)

Eczema and false food allergy

Some foods contain very powerful chemicals which exert a drug-like effect on the body. In relation to eczema, we must consider naturally occurring histamine. Foods which contain histamine, or which stimulate the release of histamine from the body's own internal stores, can cause a flare-up of eczema. To understand this clearly, just think about antihistamines for a moment — the medicines we use to treat allergies. Antihistamines work by blocking the release of histamine in the body. In so doing, they reduce itch and other symptoms. Well, here we have a group of foods which have the opposite effect: they induce itch! This happens not because you are allergic to them, but because they are laden with a very potent mediator of itch, namely histamine. These pharmacological reactions are very often dose-dependent. That is, a small dose of the food in question will cause little or no reaction, and larger doses will cause larger reactions. Most patients with eczema will therefore tolerate small amounts of histamine-containing foods. However, imagine the following histamine-rich meal. It starts off with prawn cocktail in egg mayonnaise, followed by pork with side salad of tomato, and then a plate of fresh strawberries served on a meringue base. This is washed down with a few glasses of wine. Finally, you just can't resist a nibble or two of nice chocolate. It is this sort of cumulative effect — the coincident consumption of histamine-rich foods — which is likely to bring on a flare-up of eczema. Similarly, an 'overdose' of any one of these foods is likely to cause trouble. This explains why some people get itchy at Easter: they overdose on chocolate! For full details of histamine foods and symptoms see chapter 10.

Are there any complications?

Apart from the obvious misery of constant itch, occasional infection, disrupted sleep and social embarrassment, there are two serious complications of eczema which should be noted. Both of these relate to eczema which is extensive and out of control. The first (and more subtle) complication is a failure to thrive in childhood. These children have stunted growth and must be offered urgent and effective treatment if they are to rejoin the growth curve. One can easily imagine the great drain of energy suffered by the body in trying to cope with extensive inflammation of the skin. Energy which would normally be directed towards growth is now being siphoned off to repair vast areas of damaged skin. The equivalent complication in (fully grown) adults is constant fatigue.

The second serious complication arises when the eczema flares severely and spreads to affect all or most of the body. We call this erythroderma (*erythro*: red or scalded, *derma*: skin). It is a medical emergency which requires expert help in a hospital setting to regain control.

It must be stressed that these complications are very rare, and that careful and regular attention to the underlying eczema is your best chance of avoiding them altogether.

What can we do about it?

In dealing with eczema you will want to:

1. Identify your relevant allergens and reduce your exposure to them.
2. Understand your non-allergic triggers.
3. Reduce inflammation with medication and treat complications if they arise.
4. Consider the use of nutritional supplements.
5. Consider a course of desensitisation to switch off your allergies.

Check out your allergic and non-allergic triggers

- Any child or adult with eczema which fails to respond to simple measures should be considered a candidate for the Low Allergy Diet. In children, dietary investigation should be performed only under the supervision of a medical doctor with knowledge of the subject. Adults may be able to do their own investigation by following the guidelines laid down in chapter 17.

- All patients with eczema which fails to respond to simple measures should be skin-tested for dust mite and pollen allergy.

- All patients with eczema should be aware of the list of foods which contain histamine. They may eat them in moderation, but should avoid them during times of exacerbation.

- Any late-teenager or adult with eczema which fails to respond to simple measures should be patch-tested, particularly those who have 'odd' patterns of rash, or who are at risk occupationally. (Contact allergic dermatitis is dealt with more fully in chapter 3.II.)

- Contact allergic dermatitis is not common in young children. There is, therefore, no point in patch-testing them unless they have very troublesome symptoms, or symptoms not *typical* of atopic eczema.

Other practical measures include the following:

- Nails should be kept short and clean. This will minimise

damage from scratching during sleep. If necessary, use mittens on babies' hands for the same reason.

- Clothes worn next to the skin should be pure white cotton. This is less irritating than wool and synthetic fibres. Wool is also potentially allergenic. Wash clothes in non-irritant soap.
- Baths should be restricted to a maximum of fifteen minutes. They should not be too hot because excessive heat dries the skin. Use an emollient in and immediately after the bath: pat the skin dry with a towel (no rubbing), and 'seal' the skin at once with aqueous cream or emollient, even when it is still moist from the bathwater.
- Soap and shampoo should be avoided. They have a detergent effect, taking natural oils away from the skin. Use aqueous cream and emollients instead; your doctor or chemist will advise you on the various preparations available.

Medication

The aims of medical treatment are:

1. to keep the skin moist at all times
2. to reduce inflammation
3. to keep itch to a minimum
4. to treat infection if and when it occurs

Attention to the practical measures above will help to keep the skin moist. In addition, regular application of aqueous cream or emollients will prevent drying of the skin. Apply up to four times a day if necessary. Inflammation must be controlled by the use of topical (placed directly on the skin) steroid creams or ointments. Now, I know that 'steroid' is a dirty word, and that patients (and parents) are wary of them. The decision to use a steroid treatment is based on an assessment of the likely risks and benefits to the patient. The risk of side effects from steroid creams is minimal, particularly when they are used correctly. The benefits to the patient are considerable. Furthermore, you will appreciate that the condition itself is not without risk and that withholding adequate treatment is in itself potentially dangerous.

Maureen was a case in point. She was just six years old when her parents brought her to the clinic. They were very much against the idea of using any form of medication to treat her eczema. They hoped that we could find 'the cause of it' and so avoid medication altogether. She was badly stooped as she walked into my office. She held her arms away from her tiny body, as if she had just been pulled from water, still dripping wet in all her clothes. She was unable to straighten her legs, or lift her head, because her skin was so badly inflamed. She asked if she could remain standing and explained that sitting was even more uncomfortable than her adopted pose. Her clothes were stuck to her weeping skin. One look was enough to send her straight to hospital for in-patient treatment. Her growth was stunted because her eczema had been neglected for so long, she was 'toxic' from such vast inflammation of the skin, and she was now close to serious infection. Clearly, Maureen's suffering could have been avoided by adequate treatment.

Steroids for topical application come in several strengths, ranging from mildly potent to very potent. Always use the least potent *effective* strength. Sometimes it is necessary to start with a very potent steroid to obtain control of the eczema, but this should then be scaled down to a moderately potent preparation and finally to a mildly potent one. All of these are available as creams or ointments. The former disappear more easily into the skin; the latter are greasy and are preferred if the skin is very dry or inflamed.

The itch should ultimately respond to steroid treatments. The additional use of antihistamines will help to secure a good night's sleep whilst you are waiting to gain full control, thus preventing secondary (scratch) damage to the skin. Infections are treated with antibiotics, either in topical form or as an oral preparation.

Nutritional supplements

Healthy skin is kept moist by its natural oils. These oils are called essential fatty acids (EFAs). EFAs also play a crucial role in our immune system, helping us to ward off viral infections. One would expect, therefore, that a deficiency of EFAs would lead to dry skin and frequent viral infections. This is exactly what happens in children with eczema. Indeed, some viral infections sabotage the body's utilisation of EFAs, thereby prolonging their own chances of survival. In the process, the infected patient may suffer a flare-up of eczema. An effective part of the treatment of eczema is to ensure an adequate dietary supplement of EFA in a form that viruses cannot sabotage. Gammalinolenic acid (GLA) is one such form. Good sources include evening primrose oil, starflower oil and concentrated

GLA. Studies have shown that patients with eczema who take these supplements do improve, but they may not notice the improvement until they have been on them for two to three months. It may also be worth taking a supplement of fish oil concentrate. This will provide another EFA called eicosapentenoic acid (EPA). EPA and GLA will work together to enhance the skin's natural moisture. I like to think of this as moistening the skin 'from the inside out' rather than attempting to do so 'from the outside in'.

Desensitisation

Patients who are known to be allergic to foods and/or inhalant allergens may enjoy benefit from a course of desensitisation as described in chapter 18.

Could it be anything else?

Yes. Check out the other types of dermatitis in chapter 3.II.

3.II   *Allergy and the Skin: Contact Allergic Dermatitis*

CASE HISTORY

Róisín was a 35-year-old nurse and she had developed a peculiar rash. It was odd only because of where it was: one big patch on the right side of her neck just below the ear, and another on the outer aspect of her left arm. Nowhere else was affected. The rash had been present for many months, and she had tried several creams with varying degrees of success. She was puzzled by its persistence. 'Do you always sit like that?' I asked. 'Like what?' she said. 'With your right hand tucked in under your chin one minute, and stroking the side of your left arm the next!' She did always sit like that, and when I advised her to stop wearing nail varnish, the rash disappeared. Róisín had **contact allergic dermatitis**. In her case it was an allergy to something in the nail varnish.

What is contact allergic dermatitis?

Contact allergic dermatitis, as the name suggests, refers to an allergic inflammation of skin in response to contact with an allergen: in other words, a reaction to something we touch. The reaction is a type 4 hypersensitivity: a slow and somewhat cumbersome process. It starts when allergen penetrates the skin. Small molecules penetrate further than larger ones, which is why we so readily become allergic to smaller molecules, such as nickel. Immune cells, normally resident in skin, pick up the allergen and travel with it to the lymph glands. This journey takes about twenty-four hours. These special cells then present the allergen to the immune system and ask it for judgment: do we 'tolerate' this allergen, or 'reject' it?

Certain people are genetically predisposed to reject more than they tolerate, and these are the individuals who develop contact allergic dermatitis. Their immune system sends a hostile message back to the site of original contact. Before long, they end up with a full-blown allergic inflammation in the skin. Furthermore, now that the immune system has been alerted to this allergen, it will post cells all over the body which have been programmed specifically to watch out for it. That's why a contact allergy, once established, will eventually occur wherever the allergen is placed, and not just at the site of original contact. Christine, for example, developed an itchy rash on her left wrist. Some time later she developed a similar rash on her ear lobes, and finally, by the time she came to the Allergy Clinic, she had a rash just below her navel! Christine was allergic to nickel, for she had dermatitis wherever she had contact with this allergen, namely in her watch strap, earrings and belt.

Come back now for a moment to this notion of 'original contact'. The allergen may be fixed in one spot, but immune cells are not! Thus, an allergy to the nickel in a watch strap will affect the underlying skin at the wrist, but the allergic reaction may spread up the arm as far as the shoulder! The nickel, as I say, is not moving, but the immune cells are. Now consider such migration of allergy away from the sites of watch strap, earrings, necklace, buckle and bra straps! You can imagine how easily the pattern of 'original contact' is quickly lost in this scenario. Never fear, allergy (patch) tests will reveal the truth.

Who gets it?

Contact allergic dermatitis can occur in all age groups, from early infancy to old age. However, it is far more common in young and middle-aged adults; and especially common in women — because they have greater exposure to nickel, hair colours, fragrances, cosmetics, and the like. The skin normally acts as a barrier to the outside world, but it's a barrier that can be breached. When the integrity of skin is compromised by injury or disease the breach is even greater, and larger amounts of allergen are allowed to penetrate. Thus, contact allergy occurs more readily in patients with damaged skin, such as those with eczema, other diseases of skin, and leg ulcers (see below).

Will they grow out of it?

In a word, no. But there is a curious phenomenon which has been observed in some individuals. They become allergic to something at work, continue to work with the allergen, and then for some unknown reason develop tolerance to it again. This is important for anyone considering their future in a job which involves continued contact with allergen — it might, just might, go away!

What causes it?

We can develop a contact allergy to virtually anything we touch. However, as stated above, small molecules, such as nickel, are more adept at penetrating skin. Another factor which determines our propensity for contact allergy to a given allergen is the frequency with which we come into contact with it. Patients invariably find it hard to believe that they can become allergic to something out of the blue. But it's the very handling of the allergen which predisposes to the allergy! This is most clearly seen in cases of occupational allergy, in which allergens in the workplace may be handled regularly for many years before an allergy develops.

These 'out-of-the-blue' allergies regularly occur in other settings as well. Carol, for instance, was in an awful state. Her scalp, neck and face were red, swollen and blistered. She had been to the hairdresser two weeks ago, and started to feel an ominous itch in the scalp that same night. When she woke the following morning she was horrified at what she saw in the mirror. She guessed it must have had something to do with the hairdresser. 'I thought they put too much of something in,' she said. She washed her hair again and again over the next few days, but by now she was in pain and felt sick. 'Well,' she said, 'it couldn't be an allergy because I've had this colour put in before.' 'And how did you feel the last time you had that colour?' I asked. 'A bit itchy,' she admitted, 'but only for a few days.' Carol had become allergic to the dye. The first itch was a warning unheeded, and patch tests confirmed that she was indeed highly sensitive to an ingredient of the dye.*

The list of allergens that can cause contact allergic dermatitis is truly mind-boggling. Thus, we owe a great deal of gratitude to the authoritative bodies who have pooled their knowledge and resources to give us a list of the most common culprits. We now use these when we test our patients for allergy. (See chapter 17 for a full list.)

---

*All of this agony could have been prevented if the hairdresser had followed the manufacturer's instructions: patch-test the client first.

Are there any serious complications?

Contact allergic dermatitis is, by and large, an easily treated disorder. Indeed, the most difficult aspect of treatment is to get the diagnosis right in the first place. Some patients have suffered years of discomfort because their allergy was thought to be something else. True complications are rare, although there are serious implications for those whose livelihood depends on continued contact with something they are allergic to. A young woman who cannot wear perfume is one thing; a baker who is allergic to flour is another matter entirely.

A word about contact allergic dermatitis in young children

Very young children are prone to several skin conditions, many of them unrelated to allergy. Cradle cap and nappy rash are examples. However, infants may become allergic to, or suffer irritation from, the topical creams and baby oils used to treat their skin. The contact allergy in this case resembles a 'prickly heat' rash.

Babies and older children may develop contact allergy to:

- the vinyl name-band put on them in hospital
- the clip on their name-band
- disinfectant on the thermometer
- perfumed oils, soaps and powders
- food or fruit juice — rash on their chubby cheeks
- cosmetics worn by mother — rash on the child's cheeks and forehead
- floor wax and polish — rash on hands and legs from crawling
- crayons, finger-paints, chemical sets, etc. — rash on hands and mouth
- toilet seats — rash on buttocks and thighs
- rubber — in shoes, on pencils, balloons, etc.
- bubble gum — rash around the mouth

Some of these conditions may resemble the rash of contact irritant dermatitis. For example, rubber footwear such as 'runners' or tennis shoes may cause a nasty irritation by rubbing against sweaty feet. Similarly, young girls who frequently wash their dolls' clothes may suffer an irritant dermatitis on their hands. Too many bubble baths could have the same effect.

A word about contact allergic dermatitis in the elderly

Old Mr Cole was a grumpy old soul! Seventy-five grumpy years behind him now, and not too many more to go. He was a rough sort of fellow who worked (and drank) at sea for most of his life. During his last hospital admission 'for a heart attack, or something like that' (dismissing it with a wave of his hand), he was prescribed a cream for his dry skin. 'Sure, it's weather-beaten, doctor, and I tear it at night when it's itchy.' The problem was, old Mr Cole was allergic to the cream. His arms and back were very angry — and so was he! His dry skin persisted, but he now had a raging contact allergic dermatitis wherever the cream had been lovingly applied by his long-suffering wife. Patch tests confirmed the allergy, and pinpointed exactly what it was in the cream that he had reacted to so badly. Furthermore, patch tests revealed other potential problems with contact allergens, namely fragrances. 'You wouldn't catch me dead with them things!' he said, with horror in his eyes. But what he didn't realise was that many other medicated creams contain fragrance. We were now in a position to tell his doctor which creams were safe, and which ones were not. Have you ever seen a contented grumpy old man?

Elderly skin differs from younger skin in that it loses its elasticity and its moisture. It has also been exposed, over the years, to damaging ultraviolet radiation from the sun. Consequently, elderly skin is more vulnerable to irritation, roughness, drying and damage. As we have seen, such damaged skin may now become 'supersensitive' and may react to all manner of substances, even things which we would normally consider as bland. The rash of contact allergic dermatitis, when it occurs, is also different in older skin — scaling is more prominent, the skin thickens, dark patches of pigment readily occur, and itching is intense. It is often more difficult to treat, even when the offending allergen is known.

Apart from the universal risk of contact allergy, the elderly have a few problems which are unique to their age group, and which deserve special mention. These are *stasis dermatitis*, *leg ulcers* and *occupational dermatitis*. We should also be aware that certain conditions of skin may be the presenting feature of an underlying disease (in all age groups), so if you have an undiagnosed rash, get it checked out.

Stasis dermatitis, leg ulcers and contact allergy

Some elderly patients suffer from a poor blood supply to the skin of their ankles and lower legs. This inadequate blood flow results in a skin rash which we call 'stasis dermatitis' (stasis, in this case, referring to sluggish blood flow). The skin is now at risk of breaking down altogether, to form an ulcer. As mentioned above, such a catastrophic breach of skin integrity sets one up for sensitisation. *The most common cause of contact allergic dermatitis in the elderly is a reaction to creams applied to stasis dermatitis and leg ulcers.*

We should now take a minute to consider another very important complication of stasis dermatitis. Mr O'Donnell, who was recently referred to the Allergy Clinic, is a case in point. He had developed a widespread itchy rash. It kept him awake all night, and it was driving him daft. He had been given several creams by his doctor, some of them quite strong, but he was just getting worse. He thought that sugar was aggravating his rash, and thereby assumed that he must have an allergy. However, during his initial evaluation it became quite clear that allergy was not his problem. 'Where did this rash start?' I asked him. 'Here!' he said, pulling up his trouser legs, 'And a few months later the rest of me started to itch.' He had a fulminant stasis dermatitis on both legs, and it was spreading to cover the rest of his body.

This is a potentially serious situation in which the skin of the entire body becomes severely inflamed *secondary to the stasis dermatitis.* We are not sure why this occurs, but some think it is the result of becoming allergic to one's own skin. This is how it works. The inflamed (stasis) skin is broken and damaged. The damaged skin looks different to the immune system, and elicits a hostile response from it. The immune response is clumsy. It lacks specificity. Consequently, healthy skin gets caught in the crossfire. That's why we call it 'autosensitisation' (becoming sensitised to one's self). Mr O'Donnell was sent to hospital as an emergency for treatment of his stasis dermatitis. It had become so widespread that he could now become seriously ill. He did quite well, and was discharged after a few days with ongoing treatment for his legs.

But what about his sugar allergy? It wasn't an allergy at all, it was a rationalisation! He was desperate to find a cause and a cure for his itch. In his frustration he constantly asked himself 'Could it be this?' and 'Could it be that?' His wife chirped in as well: 'I think it's "the other"' (whatever 'the other' might be). This searching is perfectly understandable, but it is frantic, and it leads to dead ends and roundabouts.

Occupation and contact allergy in the elderly
Finally, it should be noted that older patients are not exempt from other contact allergies. In particular, it is possible for the older worker to become allergic to something they have handled for many years. Builders and bakers are most at risk, but any allergen may cause similar problems. Furthermore, it may be difficult to bring the condition under control even after immediate retirement.

A word about contact allergic dermatitis in the sexually active

It is important, in the search for possible allergens, to consider the possibility that you are allergic to your partner — or at least to something *they* are wearing! Are you allergic to their perfume (or aftershave), *their* suntan lotion, *their* topical medication or *their* contraceptive? Similarly, partners have been known to react to allergens brought home on clothes, including wood dust, oils and fibreglass.

A word about contact allergic dermatitis in the workplace

Contact allergic dermatitis is the most common disease reported from the workplace. This is so because of the great number of allergens that we come into contact with on a daily basis at work. Masons, for example, may react to chrome in their cement, tilers to their grouting, painters to paint, gardeners to plants, doctors and nurses to latex gloves, homekeepers to rubber gloves, and factory workers to a host of allergens such as resins, metals, enzymes, glues and many, many more besides (see chapter 8).

What can we do about it?

First, establish the diagnosis. This is achieved by a careful clinical history and a patch test.

Who should be patch-tested?
Anyone with an undiagnosed dermatitis, or whose dermatitis is not responding to the usual treatment, should be patch-tested.

This includes patients with atopic, irritant, psoriatic or other forms of dermatitis. (See chapter 17 for details.)

Treatment of contact allergic dermatitis

Once the diagnosis is made, the only real option is avoidance of the culprit allergen. There is a good case to be made for prompt and 'aggressive' treatment in order to bring the rash under control as soon as possible. This will help to prevent new allergies developing. Topical steroid creams are the only real option here. However, make sure to check out the cream if the condition worsens or is slow to heal. You may develop contact allergy to a cream being used to treat contact allergic dermatitis!

Unfortunately, some patients, and especially the elderly, find that their contact allergy is slow to heal even after they have identified and avoided their allergen. It is possible that they are still covertly exposed to allergen, but is also possible that their disease is just plain stubborn. Perhaps they have now developed a 'primary' dermatitis, one which has assumed a life of its own.

Could it be anything else?

Yes! Contact allergic dermatitis should not be confused with:

- Contact irritant dermatitis
  This rash may be indistinguishable in appearance from allergic dermatitis. As the name suggests, it arises from contact with an irritant. Hands, for example, are frequently exposed to soap. This is a well-known irritant. Other irritants include detergents, antiseptics, polish, bleach, and even some raw foods. Patients with an active or past history of eczema are most at risk of developing an irritant dermatitis. This may be a particular source of confusion for them: they will automatically look for an allergic explanation for what appears to be a recurrence of their eczema. However, once they understand the mechanisms of irritation they will be better placed to avoid it.
- Contact urticaria
  Itchy red lumps (hives) on the skin at a site of contact. They are usually allergic in origin, and are driven by IgE. In other words they are usually a type 1 hypersensitivity reaction, and consequently are much faster to come, and to go. This could be the harbinger of more serious allergy. See chapters 3.III and 9.

- Other conditions of skin
Contact allergic dermatitis may be hard to distinguish from other diseases of skin, including fungal infection, psoriasis and other forms of dermatitis. Of special interest is the patient with psoriasis who develops a worsening of psoriasis at the site of repeated trauma: for instance, the metal sheet cutter who gets psoriasis on the palms of his hands after many months of tightly gripping the cutting tool. This may look like a contact allergy, particularly if it is accompanied by a flare-up of psoriasis elsewhere, but it's a feature of psoriasis, not allergy.

3.III   Allergy and the Skin: Hives and Swellings

(Urticaria and Angioedema)

We now turn our attention to one of the most challenging of skin conditions. We call it urticaria, and in so doing we are immediately faced with our first challenge: urticaria is not really a definitive diagnosis, it's a descriptive term. What does it describe? Hives, weals, 'nettle rash', blotches, itchy red lumps — call them what you like! They can affect part or all of the body. They are sometimes tiny, sometimes large. They may be sparse or profuse, flat or raised, round or irregular, and sometimes they produce florid and stunning patterns. Some of them disappear within the hour (only to be replaced by new ones), and others stay for days. In the most severe (and vanishingly rare) cases the patient may go into shock and die.

Urticaria is often accompanied by large swellings of the skin which we call angioedema: the result of leakage (*edema*) from blood vessels (*angio*). These swellings, in turn, are sometimes small, sometimes enormous, sometimes painful, often disfiguring, and occasionally, if they block the airway, life-threatening. The one thing that virtually all urticarias have in common is this: they are *very* itchy and *very* troublesome.

What is urticaria?

To help you understand what happens in urticaria I need to introduce you to a very special cell, the mast cell. Mast cells are found in many different parts of the body, including the lining to the nose, the chest, the eyes, the skin, the gut, etc. This widespread distribution explains, at least in part, some of the diversity of allergic symptoms. To all intents and purposes, if mast cells burst in your bronchial tubes you get asthma, in your nose you get rhinitis, in your eyes you get conjunctivitis, and so forth. Well, if they burst in your skin you get urticaria.

To say that they 'burst' is a bit crude and somewhat simplistic, but it does get the message across. Each mast cell, when viewed under the microscope, looks like a bunch of grapes. Each grape, in this analogy, represents a vesicle, or a blister. These vesicles are full of very potent chemicals, such as histamine. If and when these vesicles burst, and in so doing release their histamine, you get a hive.

To take it one step further, if they burst close to the surface of the skin you get a hive, but if they burst in the deeper layers of skin you get angioedema. That's why you often get hives and swellings together; they are one and the same event. Finally, urticaria may be either acute, lasting less than eight weeks, or chronic, persisting beyond eight weeks and sometimes for many years.

Who gets it?

Anybody can, and up to 20 per cent of the population will have experienced a bout of urticaria by the time they reach mid-life. The acute urticarias are more common in young adults with a history of allergy. The chronic varieties are more common in middle-aged women. In rare cases, it runs in families.

What causes it?

Acute urticaria

Anne was twenty-four and had never had cause to visit a doctor until now. Four weeks ago she broke out in a rash of itchy bumps. They were all over her body, and showed no sign of abating. I enquired about her recent diet, whether or not she had taken medication, where she had been, and so forth. But I could find no clues. Apart from the inconvenience of an irritating itch, she was perfectly well. I told her that she had acute urticaria: acute not in the sense that it was dangerous, but in that it was of relatively short duration. Acute urticarias come and go mysteriously, usually within six to eight weeks. I also told her that we would probably never discover the cause of her rash, and that we wouldn't have to. In all probability, it would settle within the next four weeks, and she would never be troubled by it again. Meanwhile, she should take an antihistamine to give herself some relief from itch as she awaited her spontaneous remission.

Most acute urticarias will disappear without explanation, with no clue as to what caused them, and with no particular risk of recurrence. Having said that, if you have acute urticaria ask yourself some simple questions. For example, have you recently . . .

• had an infection?	Viral, bacterial, fungal and parasitic infections may all cause urticaria. Treat the infection, the urticaria will disappear.
• taken a medicine?	Aspirin, penicillin and many others may cause urticaria. You may need to stop taking the drug because the allergy could get worse — much worse! Discuss an alternative with your doctor.
• enjoyed a dietary indiscretion?	Some foods will cause urticaria in some individuals when eaten in excess, e.g. chocolate and alcohol (see chapter 10).
• been handling . . .	citrus fruit, strawberry, fish, jellyfish, some plants, chemicals at work, etc.?
• eaten . . .	a food to which you are allergic? If you are getting acute urticaria from food, you will often notice the association yourself. The onset of symptoms will be rapid: 'Every time I eat such-and-such I get hives!'

If you cannot answer yes to any of the above, forget about it. Take an antihistamine every day and go back to the doctor if it doesn't disappear within eight weeks. Having said that, seek immediate medical help if . . .

• you have associated symptoms, such as joint pain, fever, wheeze, shortness of breath, etc.
• you have throat swelling which renders it difficult to breathe or swallow
• you are hoarse, which is a sign of laryngeal (voice box) swelling

Chronic urticaria
George was an art teacher who presented some months ago with a long history of hives and swellings. He also had an irritable bowel. This was an important clue because irritable bowel is often associated with reactions to food. It was therefore possible

that his urticaria was also food-related. He was so badly affected that he had been taking seven or eight antihistamine tablets each day in pursuit of relief. This was a very dangerous practice which he was advised to abandon forthwith. (It could have caused his heart to stop!) All of his skin tests were negative so we went straight into a Low Allergy Diet. Within seven days he had stopped itching. He was also delighted to discover that his bowel symptoms had disappeared. Unfortunately, we found that he was intolerant to many foods, far too many to avoid (and remain sane!). He was therefore started on a course of desensitisation and was doing very well. *He had chronic urticaria which was associated with multiple food intolerance.*

Poor Mrs Brennan also had chronic urticaria. In fact, she had served a nine-year 'sentence' with this dreaded itch. She assured me that she had not had a single day without symptoms during all of this time. She thought that sunlight affected her, and that she was worse just before a menstrual period. However, skin tests revealed that she was allergic to Candida, a yeast which we all have in our intestine. Within two weeks of starting anti-fungal medication she was free of itch.

Unfortunately, not all patients are so lucky. They may never find the cause of their urticaria. Kate, for instance, first presented two years ago with a similar story. Itch, itch, itch. She had chronic urticaria, there was no doubt, but try as we might, we could not find a cause for it. Okay, so what? We can't find the cause, but that doesn't mean we have to put up with it, surely! We tried the simple measures first, then the complex, then the sublime and the sophisticated. But try as we might, we made only the slightest impression on it. How frustrating!

The chronic urticarias are a real nuisance, but before we get into it let me give you one word of encouragement: there is a very high rate of spontaneous remission. In fact, there is a 50 per cent chance that your urticaria will mysteriously disappear within the next six months. However, statistics were of little value to Kate, and they may be poor consolation to you now. Nevertheless, it is important to remember this phenomenon. Why? Because if you gave up a food or a hobby, or got rid of the cat, and subsequently lost your urticaria, you may assume that your diagnosis is right, when it's wrong! Always double-check to make sure that it wouldn't have disappeared anyway.

Now for the bad news. The vast majority of chronic urticarias are 'we-don't-know-what-causes-it' urticarias. When doctors don't know the cause of something they call it 'idiopathic', and 80 to 90 per cent of chronic urticarias are thought to be idiopathic. However, a word of caution here. Mrs Brennan had idiopathic urticaria until we tracked down the cause! So, if you have chronic idiopathic urticaria *get it checked out*.

Start by keeping a diary, and don't worry if you see no pattern — this in itself would be important information. Take a glance back at the causes of acute urticaria — you may have ongoing exposure to one of these. Also note the season, the place, the activities and your diet at the time of flare-ups. Now, ask yourself these questions.

Does it happen only when I have . . .

• been vibrating?	Jerking repetitive movements can result in urticaria. For example, using kango hammers, drilling, etc.
• exercised?	It is very important to distinguish this from exercise-induced anaphylaxis (see chapter 9).
• applied pressure?	Pressure applied to the skin may result in immediate or delayed urticaria. Don't forget tight shoes, bra straps, wrist bands, etc.
• been hot?	This includes getting 'hot under the collar', labouring over the stove, hot baths or showers.
• been cold?	This includes cold air from an open car window, cold water and cold weather.
• been exposed to light?	By this we mean sunlight, whether natural or artificial.
• touched water?	Irrespective of the temperature, some people get urticaria when their skin is wet.
• been upset?	Urticaria is often a stress-sensitive condition. Mast cells have a nerve supply which can burst them in times of anger or grief.

You will notice that many of the chronic urticarias have nothing whatever to do with allergy. We call them 'physical urticarias'. Mind you, they can be just as troublesome and just as frightening as the allergic ones. Ask Pamela about that! She was a 32-year-old gymnastics teacher who recently returned from holiday with a dramatic story. She noticed a bit of an itch after swimming one day, but it soon settled down and she thought no more about it. A few days later she went for another swim and this time started to itch whilst in the sea. Within minutes she was in real trouble. She was short of breath and had a pounding headache. She was also aware that her heart was racing. She just about managed to make it back to the shore. It was then that she saw that her body was covered with 'nettle rash'. Pamela had just survived a severe episode of cold-induced urticaria. If she wants to swim in future, it will have to be in an indoor heated pool, and even then she will have to be careful.

So, as you can see, the urticarias are extremely diverse. Nevertheless, this diversity is easily explained: anything which can burst a mast cell can give you urticaria! Thus, some patients' mast cells burst when they are cooled, or heated, or pressed, or stroked, or shaken, or exposed to sunlight, etc. Similarly — and by entirely different mechanisms — they may burst when exposed to an allergen, or even as a result of emotional upset.

Will they grow out of it?

In most cases, yes. However, this will depend very much on whether the cause can be identified and avoided. Even the chronic idiopathic varieties tend to burn themselves out eventually. In some poor unfortunates it goes on and on for years.

Are there any complications?

Most urticarias are more of a nuisance than a threat. However, there is no doubt that chronic urticaria can be demoralising. It can also seriously disrupt sleep, and it can sometimes become an obsession. Indeed, some patients become more obsessed with the cause of the itch than with the itch itself! These may invest a great deal of time and money trying to get to the root of their problem, only to become increasingly frustrated by their lack of success.

In some patients, the urticaria can progress to seriously affect other systems in the body besides the skin. The symptoms which ensue are due to the direct effects of histamine release from mast cells in other parts of the body. Affected patients may complain of joint pain and abdominal pain. They may also feel feverish. Continued and more widespread histamine release may lead to fatal or near-fatal anaphylaxis. This is true not only of allergic urticaria, but of the other (physical) urticarias. To make the point, Pamela nearly died from cold-induced urticaria.

Rarely, an angioedema (swelling) may occur in the throat or voice box. Space is limited in these areas, so even moderate swellings may obstruct the airway. This happened to Imelda on her fifteenth birthday. There was great fun at the party, and junk food aplenty. Suddenly, Imelda couldn't breathe. There was absolutely no movement of air in or out of her chest. She stood slightly forward with her mouth agape and tongue protruding. Her friends looked on in horror as she turned an ominous shade of purple. One of them, who thought she was choking, came forward to slap her on the back. As her hand came down on the chest wall there was an immediate silent 'cough' of expelled air, but this was not followed by an intake of air! Imelda, of course, was terrified. She ran out of the house in desperation and fell to the ground. She had a complete airway obstruction from swelling. Fortunately, the swelling subsided of its own accord, almost as rapidly as it had developed, and Imelda was able to breathe again. She had a close call. A little detective work led us to the culprit: she was reacting to sulphites, preservatives used in some soft drinks. You will find more information on airway obstruction in chapter 7.

What can we do about it?

We can treat urticaria with medication. This is often the easiest option, just swallow the tablet(s) and get on with your life as you wait for the spontaneous remission. The medicines, when used correctly, are quite safe. The first medicine to try is an anti-histamine. If adequate doses are not working for you, your doctor may add a second medicine to the first. The rationale here is to try to stabilise mast cells so that they do not burst at the slightest whim. If this fails there are other options, but this will depend on the kind of urticaria you have. For example, beta blockers are quite good for one specific (adrenergic) kind of urticaria, but useless in others. If medication fails to give relief, or if you simply don't want to take medication for the foreseeable future, you may wish to proceed with a bit of detective work. Again, this will depend on your urticaria, your associated symptoms and your choice.

Skin-prick or patch tests do sometimes help. If a specific allergen is identified, avoid it or kill it (anti-fungals). If these tests draw a blank, move on to dietary manipulations. There are two diets that may be of help:

1. The Low Allergy Diet (described in chapter 17) is worth considering, *particularly if you have other symptoms of food allergy or intolerance.*
2. The Low Salicylate Diet is also worth considering, *particularly if you are allergic to aspirin, and/or if you suffer from rhinitis, asthma or nasal polyps.* This diet will get rid of some 30 per cent of urticarias. It's a bit of a pain in the neck, but then so is living with an intractable itch!

The Low Salicylate Diet

Salicylates are naturally occurring substances that can cause 'allergic' reactions, including rhinitis, asthma, nasal polyps, urticaria, and hyperactivity (in children). Aspirin is salicylic acid, one of the salicylates. If you have any of the allergic conditions mentioned above, and particularly if you are allergic to aspirin, you may benefit from a diet which excludes naturally occurring salicylates. You will need to stick to the diet for one month in the first instance.

The following foods are high in salicylate and should be avoided:

- most herbs and spices
- most fruit, but see below
- most vegetables, but see below
- most nuts
- coffee and tea
- Coca-Cola and peppermint tea
- fruit juices (except the fruits mentioned below)
- alcoholic drinks — but gin and vodka might be okay
- honey, liquorice and peppermint
- Marmite, Bovril, stock cubes and yeast-rich products
- tomato and Worcester sauce
- processed foods and instant meals — preservatives, colourings, flavourings, etc.

The following are low in salicylate, and may be eaten ad lib:

- meat — all kinds
- fish — all kinds
- milk, cheese and eggs
- wheat, rye, barley and rice
- allowed fruit: banana, peeled pear, lemon, pomegranate, papaya, passion fruit and mango
- allowed vegetables: cabbage, Brussels sprouts, bean sprouts, celery, leeks, lettuce and peas; potato skins are high, but the potato itself is okay
- miscellaneous allowed: carob, cocoa, cashew nut

Also stay away from aspirin, and any medicine which contains aspirin. Non-steroidal anti-inflammatory drugs (NSAIDs) should also be avoided. Salicylate symptoms should disappear within one month of this diet. Try expanding it at that stage to see what you can get away with. Please get advice if you stay on this or any other diet for longer than one month.

Could it be anything else?

Urticaria should not be confused with:

- insect bites (midges, fleas, bedbugs, lice, etc.)
- scabies
- other diseases. Sometimes urticaria is part and parcel of another disease, such as hepatitis, lupus or others. A good clinical history together with a physical examination and a few simple blood tests will allow your doctor to rule these out.

But I get an itch without a rash!

Generalised itch may represent an underlying disease or a skin disease — even in the absence of a visible rash. Check it out with your doctor; meanwhile watch out for:

- scabies
- lice
- contact with fibreglass: this may cause itch before a rash
- contact with wool, hairs, plant spicules, fabric softeners, anti-static laundry products
- visiting insects: fleas, animal scabies, other mites
- low humidity of heated air, or air-conditioned air in summer, which can contribute to dryness of skin and itch
- some prescribed medicines!

4 *Allergy in the Nose and Sinuses*

The healthy nose and sinuses

The nose has an important protective function for the respiratory tract. It stands like a sentinel at a gate. It serves to moisten and filter inspired air. The nose is also called upon to handle more infectious agents than any other organ in the body. This 'air-conditioning' effect ensures that the air reaching the bronchial tubes and lungs is at its most suitable. Much of this gatekeeper function is performed by special structures in the nose called turbinates. These are sausage-shaped bones with a very rich, blood-filled lining. There are three of them in each nostril. They go through cycles of periodic congestion and decongestion, first expanding with blood (congestion), and then contracting (decongestion), washing away filtered debris in the process. For the most part we are completely unaware of this action, but if we do become aware of it, one nostril may feel obstructed when it isn't. You can test this out on your own nose as you read. Block one nostril gently with a finger and breathe through the other nostril; you will find that one nostril feels 'more open' than the other. Try again later, and the opposite will occur.

The nostrils are separated from each other by a partition of cartilage called the nasal septum. Between the turbinates and the septum there is very little free space. This should be considered a deliberate design feature because larger spaces would result in less efficient air-conditioning.

The sinuses are hollow (air-filled) spaces within the bones surrounding the nose. Thus, there are sinuses in the cheekbones (the maxillary sinuses), in the bones above the eyes (the frontal sinuses), and in the bones between the eyes (the ethmoidal sinuses). All of these drain into and are continuous with the nasal cavity. For this reason, the nose and the sinuses should be considered together: they are one organ. Finally, the nasal cavity is also connected to (and receives drainage from) the middle ear by means of a duct called the Eustachian tube.

There is a price to pay for such sophistication in a limited space, and it's this. Narrow spaces are quickly blocked. Thus, even a slight deformity of the nasal septum, a small polyp or any degree of inflammation in the nose will quickly produce symptoms of nasal obstruction. Obstructions, wherever they occur in the body, frequently lead to infection. Thus an obstructed Eustachian tube, for example, can lead to an infection of the middle ear. Similarly, obstruction of sinus drainage points will lead to infection in the sinus. We refer to these infections as secondary phenomena: secondary, that is, to obstruction.

CASE HISTORY

Ciara is a ten-year-old girl. 'She has had one cold after another for the past two years,' her mother said. I asked her what she meant by that. 'She is always getting sore throats and sore ears, she sniffs all the time, and she can't breathe through her nose,' she explained. The child was the portrait of misery. 'And look!' she continued, pointing to the girl's upper lip, 'She has the skin of her face rubbed raw with tissues.' It did not take long to hazard a guess at the problem: the lining inside Ciara's nose was inflamed. It looked an angry blood-red. There was also a copious nasal discharge of clear mucus, like raw egg white. Her turbinates were swollen to the point of obstructing both nostrils. She was breathing through her mouth. In addition, one ear was full of fluid, as could be seen through a lacklustre eardrum. Skin tests revealed that Ciara was highly allergic to house dust mites, grass pollen and some moulds. Ciara has, until proven otherwise, an **allergic rhinitis**.

What is allergic rhinitis?

Allergic rhinitis refers to an inflammation of the lining of the nose caused by allergy (*rhin-*, as in rhinoceros!). The symptoms include:

- 'runny' nose (rhinorrhoea)
- sneezing, usually in bouts of several or many sneezes
- itchy nose
- itch of the soft palate (the 'roof' at the back of the mouth)
- itchy ears
- nasal obstruction

There is nothing half-hearted about the inflammation of allergic rhinitis. The normally neat and tidy lining of the nose becomes packed with cells migrating in from the bloodstream. These are immune cells, and they have been summoned to the site by an 'allergic call'. Special cells in the nose, called mast cells, have burst because they have been touched by something they are allergic to. When they burst, their contents (highly active chemicals) spill out into the surrounding tissues. This is the first step in the 'allergic cascade'. These chemicals are responsible for the first symptoms of allergy: namely, itch, sneezing and a runny nose. They are also the 'SOS' by which other cells are called to battle. As these cells crowd into the narrow spaces of the nasal cavity, they cause obstruction. Thus, obstruction is a later symptom of allergy.

Who gets it?

Allergic rhinitis is very common. Some 10 per cent of children and 30 per cent of adolescents are affected. However, it is also possible to develop the condition in early infancy or at any stage in adulthood, including old age. In general, the older you are before you first develop rhinitis, the less likely it is to be allergic in origin (see below for a word on non-allergic rhinitis).

Will they grow out of it?

Allergic rhinitis is usually a long-term disorder, with patients suffering symptoms over many years. Symptoms will fluctuate depending on exposure to allergen, weather, etc. Occasionally there is a spontaneous remission, but don't hold your breath waiting for one!

What causes it?

Allergic rhinitis is usually caused by an allergy to something in the air we breathe. Because they are inhaled, we refer to them as 'inhalant allergens'. Less commonly, the problem is an allergy to food, or to an allergen encountered at work.

Causes of allergic rhinitis:

1. inhalant allergens
    * pollen: grass, tree and weed
    * house dust mites
    * mould spores
    * animal dander and feathers

2. ingested allergens
   • food and drink
3. occupational allergens

1. Inhalant allergens

The pattern of your symptoms depends entirely on what you are allergic to. For example, if you are allergic to grass pollen you will have symptoms only when significant amounts of grass pollen are in the air. Your symptoms will start towards the end of May and continue throughout the summer, gradually decreasing towards the end of August. Similarly, if you were allergic to tree pollen, or weed pollen, you would have symptoms in spring or autumn respectively.

The following table shows the more common airborne allergens in relation to the calendar. You will notice that mould, like dust mite, is a perennial allergen (present all the year round).

The perennial and seasonal nature of common allergens

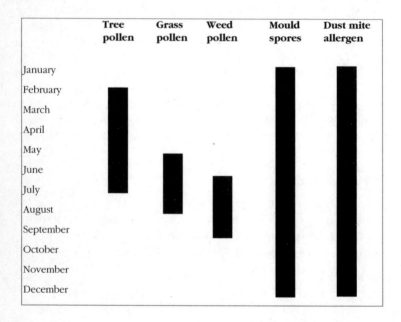

A word about 'hay fever'

Hay fever is the common name for seasonal allergic rhinitis. The symptoms are those of allergic rhinitis with the addition of itchy and watering eyes (allergic conjunctivitis); the eyes may become quite swollen and painful. Furthermore, these symptoms may be accompanied by cough, wheeze and shortness of breath. We refer to this as 'hay asthma'. Although we relate these symptoms to hay, they could just as easily be brought on by any other air-borne allergen. Interestingly, hay fever, like all allergic conditions, is becoming much more common. The first case was described in 1812, and it took doctors twelve years to collect the next twenty cases!

Not all 'seasonal' allergies are due to seasonal allergens. In one well-documented case, a young boy was told he had 'hay asthma' because he developed wheeze every summer, and specifically during the hottest, driest days of summer. He had virtually no wheeze at other times of the year. One clever fellow then spotted the fact that the young lad's wheeze was related more to his ingestion of diluted orange drink, of which he con-sumed considerable amounts during hot summer days. The drink was laden with tartrazine, a colouring agent. He stopped drinking his tartrazine, and his 'hay' asthma disappeared for good.

A word about silver birch pollen

Silver birch pollen deserves special mention. It becomes air-borne in early spring, sometimes as early as January, and may cause a rash in allergic individuals. Thus, these patients get all the symptoms of 'hay fever' but also suffer a crop of hives (urticaria). We call this full collection of symptoms 'silver birch pollenosis'. There is another aspect to silver birch allergy which is quite fascinating: up to 60 per cent of those who are allergic to it will get a tingling sensation of the lips and tongue when they eat apple. This is what we call 'cross-reactivity'. The immune system obviously thinks that the birch and apple aller-gens are one and the same thing. Silver birch also cross-reacts in this way with parsnip, potato, carrot and hazelnut (although these do not necessarily cause tingling lips). This is reminiscent of the Oral Allergy Syndrome, in which some individuals react to almost all fruit and vegetable (see chapter 7).

A word about house dust mites and mould

As you can see, allergy to airborne pollen is a very seasonal affair. Symptoms come and go with the pollen. House dust mite allergy, on the other hand, is quite different. Symptoms are perennial, because our exposure to the mite is perennial. Symptoms may lessen somewhat during the summer, and worsen somewhat during winter, but this only reflects our lesser or greater exposure to the allergen. Mould is similar — or rather, moulds (plural) are similar. No sooner has one species quietened down than another starts to throw its spores into the atmosphere. The end result is that we are virtually constantly exposed to mould spores of one species or another.

A word about chemicals

Patients with allergic rhinitis often complain that chemical smells (such as tobacco smoke, perfumes, deodorants, etc.) aggravate their symptoms. They may then assume they are allergic to the chemicals themselves. However, most of these are irritant reactions. That is, they irritate an already inflamed nose. Treat the underlying allergy, and you will not be bothered by occasional chemical smells. In dealing with occupational allergy you will see the need to differentiate between allergic and irritant reactions, because it is, after all, possible to be allergic to chemicals as well.

2. Ingested allergens

Rhinitis and food allergy

It is very rare for an allergy to an *ingested* food to cause rhinitis without also causing some other allergic symptom. However, food *dust* can cause rhinitis with or without other symptoms. So, if you have rhinitis together with other symptoms, and if your skin tests are negative to airborne allergens, you should consider the possibility of a food allergy. The Low Allergy Diet is the only reliable test available to you for this purpose (see chapter 17).

Rhinitis and false food allergy

Bear in mind that . . .

- the act of chewing hot or spicy foods can cause the nose to 'run'
- alcohol produces nasal congestion
- caffeine can cause rhinitis: sneezing, watering and nasal obstruction

Rhinitis and aspirin sensitivity

There is another interesting cause of rhinitis: sensitivity to aspirin. This is not an allergy in the true sense of the word, because it does not involve IgE, the allergy antibody. One clue to aspirin sensitivity is, of course, a sudden worsening of symptoms immediately after taking some! However, some 25 per cent of our foods contain salicylates, substances very similar to aspirin (salicylic acid). An aspirin-sensitive patient is therefore frequently and innocently exposed to these in their everyday diet. Aspirin sensitivity is often manifested by the concurrent presence of rhinitis, polyps, hives and asthma! If you have any *three* of these conditions, follow the Low Salicylate Diet detailed on p. 49–50. An improvement in some or all symptoms would suggest that you are indeed sensitive to salicylates.

3. Occupational rhinitis

It is possible to develop rhinitic (and other) symptoms from inhalation of an allergen or irritant encountered at work, or in the course of a hobby.

Examples include:

- meal (bakers and millers allergic to wheat and rye 'dust')
- wood dusts (oak, rosewood, teak, mahogany, pine, western red cedar, etc.)
- grain (contains many different allergens including pollen, mould, storage mites, etc. Corn appears to be a particular problem in this regard.)
- enzymes (in laboratories)
- anhydrides (plastics and epoxy resins)
- latex (medical/paramedical gloves, rubber industry)

You will find much more detailed information on occupational allergies in chapter 8. Meanwhile, here's an example of what can happen at work. James, a 35-year-old haulier, complained of being 'caught in the chest': 'Not all the time, doctor, but on and off, over the past ten years or so.' He could not see a pattern to his symptoms, but when he was pressed on details, a very clear picture emerged. His first symptom would always be a 'lump in the throat'. This would be quickly followed by a runny nose with bouts of sneezing. Finally, the wheeze would start up. He had 'always put it down to a cold', and never paid that much heed to his symptoms. He was a hardy bloke, more annoyed with the inconvenience than anything else. 'What do you carry in the truck?' I asked. 'Animal feeds,' he said. 'You know, soy bean and other grains.' We arranged to skin-test him to these, and yes, he was highly sensitive to them. He was started on a programme of desensitisation, together with some medication to carry him through the rough patches. He was also careful to wear a mask when handling his loads. After a few months of treatment he was very much improved. The last time I saw him for review he told me that he had no symptoms worth talking of, 'except for a cold which started last week'. However, when we looked at his nasal discharge under the microscope it was full of allergic cells. It was clear that James was still being accidentally exposed to a relevant allergen from time to time.

Are there any complications?

At first glance, the symptoms of allergic rhinitis may not appear unduly troublesome, and may even be trivialised. However, they do have a significant effect on a patient's quality of life. Apart from the obvious discomfort and social embarrassment of the rhinitic symptoms themselves, patients must also endure:

- the secondary effects of sleep disturbance:
  — impairment of concentration
  — mood changes
  — fatigue
  — headache
- the secondary effects of nasal obstruction:
  — recurrent sinus infections
  — recurrent sore throats
  — recurrent ear problems

Let's take a closer look at Ciara's symptoms, the young girl we met earlier in this chapter. The inflammation in her nose was causing rhinorrhoea and obstruction. The obstruction was block-ing one of her Eustachian tubes, allowing an accumulation of fluid in the middle ear on that side. The resultant pressure in her ear was painful. Nasal obstruction was also causing her to breathe through her mouth, and this was drying her throat excessively, particularly during sleep. It was no wonder she had sore throats. Furthermore, because she couldn't breathe easily, her sleep was bound to be disrupted, contributing to her tired-ness and misery.

Rhinitis and asthma

There is also a direct link between rhinitis and asthma. In fact, there may even be two links. In the first place, there is a nervous connection between the nose/sinuses and the bronchial tubes. Irritation of the former may spark off an asthmatic reaction in the latter. Secondly, untreated allergic rhinitis results in the inspiration of poor-quality air. With the nose blocked, air is taken in through the mouth, and thus escapes the normal conditioning that would occur in the healthy nose. The air reaching the lungs is therefore relatively dry. It is also polluted with microscopic particles of dust and other allergens. This is not good for asthma. It is therefore important to treat rhinitis (if it is present) when treating asthma.

Rhinitis and polyps

Rhinitis is often complicated by nasal polyps. These are grape-like structures which 'grow' like a grape on a stalk. The stalk is usually out of sight, high up inside the nose. The body of the polyp may become quite large, large enough to push the sides of the nostrils out, giving the nose a swollen and deformed appearance. The problem with polyps is that they quickly cause obstruction. Even small ones strategically placed can block a sinus. Once again, obstruction leads to infection. Topical application of steroid may help to shrink the polyp(s), but surgical removal is often necessary. Polyps tend to recur, so make sure to treat the underlying allergies aggressively.

Rhinitis and other allergies

Finally, patients with allergic rhinitis (and asthma), as a group, are more likely to develop allergies to food (see chapter 7).

What can we do about allergic rhinitis?

In treating allergic rhinitis you will want to:

1. Identify your relevant allergens and reduce your exposure to them.
2. Understand your non-allergic triggers.
3. Reduce nasal inflammation with medication.
4. Treat complications if and when they occur.
5. Consider a course of desensitisation to switch off your allergies.

Check out the allergies!

The most helpful investigation for the patient with rhinitis is a detailed clinical history together with physical examination of the nose and a series of skin-prick tests. This will give very reliable information on allergy to airborne allergens. Allergens commonly tested by skin-prick test include house dust mite, pollens, moulds and animal danders. Once you know which allergens are causing your trouble you can take measures to reduce your exposure to them. The most common culprit by far is the house dust mite. If you are allergic to this allergen you would be well advised to follow the avoidance measures outlined in appendix 1.

Medical treatment for rhinitis

1. Nasal decongestants
   - Are to be avoided at all costs (see below).
   - Having said that, they may be used for a few days at the start of treatment to allow topical steroid into the otherwise blocked nose.

2. Antihistamines
   - Will reduce the immediate symptoms of allergy (itch, runny nose, sneezing and itchy eyes).
   - With one notable exception (Zirtek), they will have no effect whatever on the late symptoms of allergy, namely blocked nose.
   - Are now available over the counter in your pharmacy. Ask for a non-sedating one!

3. Topical nasal steroid sprays
   - Are quite effective.
   - Are quite safe.
   - Must be continued for at least *two weeks* before you decide that they have not worked for you.
   - Must be taken *every day* for best effect, irrespective of symptoms.

4. Intramuscular steroid injections
   - Remain an option for patients with severe disease not responsive to the above.
   - May be considered in patients facing important events, e.g. exams, weddings, etc.

5. Desensitisation
   - My preferred option; see chapter 18.

Could it be anything else?

Yes! Not all that sneezes is an allergy!

- Infective (viral) rhinosinusitis
  The majority of upper respiratory infections are 'common colds' caused by the human rhinovirus and coronavirus. These viruses force their way into the cells of the nasal mucosa and, in so doing, provoke a full inflammatory (immune) response against them. Fortunately, they are self-limiting infections, unable to sustain themselves beyond a few days. Such viral infections are very common in childhood, with perhaps even as many as five or six per year in the younger child. We need to stress this point: 'colds' are never *constant.* On the contrary, they are *self-limiting* bouts of illness, lasting no more than a few days at a time. Antibiotics, incidentally, have absolutely no effect on viruses. There is, therefore, no point in giving yourself (or little Johnny) an antibiotic for the common cold.

- Infective (bacterial) rhinosinusitis
  Sometimes bacteria take advantage of the chaos and obstruction caused by a virus. These 'superimposed' or 'secondary' bacterial infections are more troublesome and often require antibiotic treatment. Patients with untreated allergic rhinitis are at risk of recurrent bacterial infections for the same reason. Adequate treatment of the underlying allergy will greatly reduce this risk. Some unfortunate patients suffer from recurrent bacterial infections of the nose and sinuses *which we cannot explain.* Some of these may benefit from a course of treatment aimed at improving their immune function.

- Non-infective, non-allergic rhinitis (NINAR)
  This is wonderfully named! It's an 'I-don't-know-what-causes-it' rhinitis, but 'I know it's not infection and I know it's not allergy!' Having said that, we know that the nerves supplying the nasal mucosa are in overdrive. They are the force behind the inflammation, but why they do this is a mystery. We also know that it's related to age: the older you are when you first get rhinitis, the more likely it is to be non-allergic. It is in many ways a diagnosis of exclusion: we have excluded infection, and we have excluded allergy, therefore we call it NINAR. The symptoms, however, are indistinguishable from (and just as troublesome as) allergy.

- **Watch out for** . . . the side effects of medication. Some pre-scribed medicines cause rhinitis! They may do so without any other clue that you are 'allergic' to them. Check the list to make sure that you are not taking one. If you are, discuss an alternative prescription with your doctor.

  Medicines that can cause rhinitis:

  Reserpine
  Guanethidine
  Hydralazine
  Beta blockers
  Methyldopa
  ACE inhibitors
  Prazosin
  Phentolamine
  Aspirin and other non-steroidals
  Oral contraceptives
  Nasal decongestants

- **Watch out for** . . . nasal decongestants. Another fairly com-mon problem relates to the use of nasal decongestant sprays and drops. What often happens is that a patient with rhinitis first starts to use the decongestant during a time of particu-larly troublesome symptoms. They enjoy great relief from nasal obstruction (because they induce a semi-permanent contraction of their turbinates). However, once the effect of the decongestant wears off, there is a rebound swelling of the turbinates which makes the nose feel very uncomfortable. More decongestant will now provide immediate relief, but our patient is 'hooked'. To get out of this trap, use a topical nasal steroid as follows.

  Breaking the 'addiction' to nasal decongestants:

  — Apply a topical nasal steroid (on prescription from your doctor) to each nostril every morning and evening throughout the withdrawal phase.
  — Continue to use the decongestant as before.
  — After two weeks, stop using the decongestant in one nos-tril, and expect some discomfort/obstruction in this nostril for a few days.
  — Continue to apply decongestant to the other nostril as before, and the steroid spray to both nostrils.

— After a further week, stop using decongestant altogether. Again, expect some discomfort in the second nostril for a few days. Continue to apply the steroid spray to both nostrils.

— Thereafter, treat your rhinitis appropriately.

- **Watch out for** . . . female hormones. Nasal obstruction and watery nose may occur during pregnancy, particularly during the second and third trimesters. Symptoms usually resolve shortly after delivery. Patients known to have allergic rhinitis before pregnancy may notice an improvement *or* a worsening of symptoms during pregnancy. Rhinitis may also occur during or shortly after the menopause. Many women also complain that their rhinitis (and asthma) are harder to control in the premenstrual time. All of these phenomena are hormonal in nature. It is not surprising then that women on the oral contraceptive pill are also at risk of developing rhinitis: another 'hormonal rhinitis' which will resolve off the pill.

- **Watch out for** . . . other diseases. Very rarely, rhinitis may be a prominent symptom of underlying disease such as an underactive thyroid gland or Wegener's granulomatosis.

Hay fever advice

If you suffer from grass pollen allergy, follow these measures to reduce your symptoms:

1. Keep yourself informed by monitoring pollen counts:
   - Symptoms start when pollen counts reach 50 per cubic metre.
   - Symptoms are severe when counts reach 300 per cubic metre.
   - Pollen counts exceed 4,000 per cubic metre in hay fields!
   - Towards the end of the grass pollen season, you will find that even low pollen counts (*c.*30 per cubic metre) cause you trouble. This is because your system has been 'primed' by ongoing exposure to pollen over the summer months.

2. Stay indoors when counts are high:
   - Counts are highest on dry windy days.
   - Counts are highest in the afternoon and late evening because of thermal air movements.

3. Avoid high-pollen areas:
   - Holiday by the sea! Air that has travelled overland is laden with pollen; air from the sea is not.

4. Shower and change clothes as soon as you come indoors:
   - This will wash the sticky pollen away from your body.

5. Travel with windows closed, ideally in a car with pollen filtration.

6. Wear sunglasses.

7. If you wish, you could wear a special cap with face screen and air filter.

8. Use medication wisely:
   - antihistamines
     — as described above
   - topical steroid spray
     — must be started two weeks before the pollen season starts, and
     — continued throughout the season
   - eye drops for allergy (on prescription)
     — are very safe
     — are fast-acting
     — are very effective for eye symptoms
     — may be used as and when you have symptoms

9. Consider desensitisation.
   - This is my preferred option; see chapter 18.
   - You must have one injection at least four weeks before the grass pollen season starts.
   - It will increase your 'resistance' to pollen.
   - It may reduce symptoms entirely for the whole season.
   - It may also greatly reduce your need for the medications listed above.

5   Allergy and the Chest: Asthma

Healthy lungs

Have you noticed that we never think about breathing until it becomes difficult? It all happens automatically. In health, our brain sends a subconscious message to the muscles of the chest: 'Inhale!' The muscles contract and air comes rushing in. As we have seen in the previous chapter, the air is conditioned as it passes through the nose. This ensures that only filtered, warm and moist air is allowed beyond this point. The air then passes through the throat into the lower airways: the voice box, the windpipe and the bronchial tubes, and finally it reaches the lungs themselves.

The voice box, or larynx, lies in the neck. You can feel its Adam's apple halfway between your chin and your chest. It is more prominent in males, giving them a deeper voice. The windpipe, or trachea, runs from the larynx into the chest and divides into two large branches. One branch, or bronchus, goes off towards the right lung, and the other goes to the left. These in turn divide into smaller and smaller branches and twigs, much like the pattern of a tree. The air passes through these tubes and eventually comes to its final destination: microscopic air sacs called alveoli. These are the working units of the lung. In fact, these *are* the lungs! This is where it all happens, where carbon dioxide is released from the blood into the sacs, and oxygen supplies are drawn from the sacs into the blood.

If these individual alveoli were laid down side by side (instead of all grouped together into two lungs) they would cover seventy square metres — that's slightly larger than a squash court! This gives some indication of the capacity and industry of the lungs. Once the gases are exchanged, the muscles of the chest wall are allowed to relax and the used air is exhaled. Some debris from the outside world will have escaped filtration in the nose and will stick to the lining of the bronchial tree. However, the lining is equipped with tiny wafting hairs and these methodically carry debris back towards the larynx. When enough dirt accumulates, a cough reflex is initiated and the dirt is expelled from the airways. This self-cleaning capacity is limited and can be easily overcome by pollution, such as traffic fumes and tobacco smoke.

Now, imagine for a moment that you suddenly run to catch a bus. By the time you get there you're out of breath. You take your seat, puffing and panting, and you're slightly embarrassed. Thankfully, you have a bus pass to wave at the conductor — you wouldn't have the breath to tell him where you're going! You (should) think to yourself, 'I'm not fit, I really should get back to the gym.' Anyway, the puffing and panting is all automatic, driven by a specialised group of cells in the brain. These can tell whether you have enough oxygen or not. When the respiratory centre is satisfied that you have now done enough puffing and panting, it will reduce its drive, and the breathing will return to its resting state. Throughout the day, and less dramatically, our breathing will increase and decrease in this manner, depending on physical (and mental) activity. During the night, when our bodies slow down in sleep, the breathing slows down too. It reaches its 'lowest' point at about 4 a.m. But something goes wrong in asthma.

Case history

Adrian is a thirteen-year-old boy who loves sport. He has suffered from asthma since early childhood. He was taking three different inhalers every day, and was still getting symptoms. Moreover, he was waking up in the early hours of the morning for 'a few more puffs' of his inhaler. When things got out of hand, and they did several times a year, he needed oral steroid tablets. In addition, he occasionally had really bad attacks requiring admission to hospital. These were mostly associated with infection. His family doctor wondered whether there was an allergic aspect to his asthma and referred him to the Allergy Clinic. Adrian said that he manages to get by if he 'takes things easy'. But he was a sportsman, and did not want a sedentary lifestyle. He was very frustrated by his inability to run without coughing and wheezing. Taking his inhaler before a football match did not help. He also had hay fever — and a cat!

Skin tests revealed that he was highly allergic to many airborne allergens, including pollens, dust mites and moulds. He was also allergic to the cat. The first job was to clean up his home environment. He went to town on this, and adopted comprehensive allergen avoidance measures (see appendix 1). He asked someone else to adopt the cat. His asthma improved within weeks, but he still had some way to go. We then started a course of desensitisation. By the time of his fourth dose, his lung function had improved considerably, he was sleeping through the night, he played football for the school team, and he had enjoyed a summer without hay fever. We are now weaning him off his inhalers.

What is asthma?

Asthma is a chronic disorder of the airways, and as old as history itself. The Chinese Yellow Emperor, Huang Di (2697–2598 BC) is said to have referred to it; Egyptians mentioned it in the Ebers papyrus; Hippocrates thought it was caused by something in the environment; and Pliny the Elder had cases induced by pollen! We have inherited the Greek description: asthma meaning 'to pant' or 'to breathe hard'.

In a nutshell, asthma is an inflammatory condition of the bronchial tubes which makes them 'hyper-reactive'. By this we mean two things. In the first place, the bronchial tubes are *always* (chronically) inflamed, *even in cases of very mild or episodic asthma*. Secondly, the inflamed airways are very sensitive to change. They are twitchy, if you like, and they very easily overreact to environmental stimuli. When they do overreact, they go into spasm and become even more inflamed. Here again, the mast cell plays an important role. The sequence of events is easily understood.

1. The lining of the bronchial tubes becomes inflamed and swollen.
2. The inflamed lining secretes thick mucus into the airway.
3. The muscle surrounding the bronchial tubes gets twitchy and goes into spasm.

Each step in this process is marked by a further reduction in the bore (size) of the airways. Think of it like this. You're in a movie, and you're on the run from an enemy. He's armed, you're not. You come to a river, too wide to cross in a hurry. You turn around and see the bad guy in hot pursuit, so you jump in and hide amongst the bulrush. Fortunately, the director hands you a length of hosepipe, and you slip underwater breathing through the pipe. All goes well until the director decides that a drinking straw would have more dramatic effect. He makes the switch. You now have to breathe through a much smaller bore. Not only do you have to suck the air in with much greater force but you have to blow it out forcibly. Breathing is much more difficult. This is what happens in asthma: you're being asked to breathe through a smaller airway.

The symptoms of asthma are the direct result of inflamed and constricted airways. Patients experience:

1. difficulty breathing/shortness of breath
   and/or
2. tightness in the chest
   and/or
3. wheeze
   and/or
4. cough

Although most patients will experience all of these symptoms, many will not. Indeed, some patients may complain of only one symptom, such as a chronic cough, or fatigue. That's one to watch out for — a cough that just won't go away, or that goes away during the day and comes back at night. *Anyone who has a cough lasting more than four weeks should be checked out for asthma.* Don't wait for the wheeze, it may never come!

Mr Dunne was an interesting case. He was sixty-two years old and complained of fatigue. Nothing very specific, just a loss of energy. It came on him gradually over the past two years or so. Yes, he did feel a bit depressed, and yes, he was rather fed up at work. He looked forward to retirement but couldn't imagine being able to do anything with his time. The only abnormality on examination was the presence of a wheeze in his chest. He couldn't hear it, and I couldn't hear it without the stethoscope, but he had a wheeze. A few more simple tests confirmed that he had asthma. Within one month of starting treatment with two inhalers he felt much better, a return of the old sparkle! Fatigue may be the only symptom of asthma.

Who gets it?

Anybody can get asthma. It can start at any age, but more commonly in childhood, and particularly in children under the age of five years. In this age group, boys are affected twice as often as girls, possibly because they have smaller airways to begin with. However, by the age of ten years, the girls have caught up. When asthma appears for the first time in adult life, men and women are equally affected.

A lot has been said in recent years about the fact that asthma seems to be on the increase. However, those who have studied the details give conflicting reports, ranging from 'little increase' to '500 per cent increase'. The truth probably lies somewhere between these two extremes, but there is no doubt about it: asthma is becoming more common, and there are now an estimated 100 million people worldwide with the condition. Finally, certain occupations may put you at risk, so have a read of chapter 8.

Will they grow out of it?

In a word, maybe! Up to 50 per cent of affected children do seem to grow out of their asthma completely. Asthma appearing for the first time in adult life tends to be more persistent.

What causes it?

We don't know the cause of asthma, but we do know many of the 'triggers' — the things that set it off. Many of these are allergic in nature, but others are not. We also know that asthma runs in families. Specifically, it is the genetic tendency towards allergy which puts the child at risk for asthma (but not all allergic children get it). There is also an association between the risk of getting asthma and . . .

- environmental pollution (outdoor and indoor)
- tobacco smoke
- having other allergies
- being of small size at birth
- exposure to lots of allergen in the first year of life

Asthma — the allergic triggers

The allergic triggers of asthma include:

1. inhalant allergens
   - house dust mites

- pollen: grass, tree and weed
- mould spores
- animal danders: horse, cat, dog, etc.
- feathers
- others

2. ingested allergens
   - food and drink
   - food and drink additives
   - Some medicines can give us asthma. Beta blockers and aspirin are two very important examples. Talk to your doctor if you are taking one of these and your asthma is not controlled.
3. occupational allergens
   - numerous

1. A few examples of asthma triggered by inhalant allergy

James was eight years old when he first came to the Allergy Clinic. His history is quite classical and demonstrates much of what you have just read. In the first place, he came from an allergic family. His mother and several cousins had a history of hay fever. He himself had a history of eczema as a baby, but this had cleared up long ago. 'He's sneezing and wheezing!' his father said. 'And he coughs. Boy, does he cough, especially at night when we're all trying to sleep.' He was taking the usual inhalers but still getting into trouble. Like most asthmatic children, he got a bit of a wheeze when he ran about. His father, unfortunately, was a chain-smoker, and this was sure to make things worse. Skin-prick tests showed that James was allergic to the ubiquitous house dust mite, and had a lesser sensitivity to silver birch pollen. His father promised to smoke only in the back garden, and he took careful note of the measures required to reduce the dust mite allergen in James's bedroom. The boy then had one dose of desensitisation and improved so dramatically that his mother thought he was 'cured'! However, it wore off after a few months (as expected) and he is now well into his course of jabs and on the road to more permanent relief. *Asthma is often triggered by the house dust mite!*

Declan was a businessman in his late thirties. He had asthma as a young lad for a few years and then grew out of it. However, it came back to him last autumn, together with the symptoms of rhinitis. It wasn't particularly bad, he said, more of a nuisance than anything else. Again, skin tests confirmed his allergy to dust mites. He had no other allergy. Desensitisation brought about a great improvement. The last time I saw him for a booster dose he told me that he had stopped his inhalers altogether. *Asthma in adults can also be triggered by house dust mites!*

Helen is a university student coming up to her summer exams. She is 'really fed up today' because she has asthma. In fact, she tells me that she gets asthma at this time every year, and it interferes with her study. She also gets the other symptoms of hay fever. Once the summer holidays are over, she has no asthma. Skin tests confirm her allergy to grass pollen, and the fact that she is not allergic to other allergens. She has 'hay asthma'. *Asthma is sometimes triggered by seasonal allergens!*

Nuala is a housewife and mother of two. She has been very unwell in recent years with asthma. She also had repeated sinus and chest infections. Furthermore, she was admitted to hospital on two occasions with pneumonia, and once to have her nasal polyps removed. Not surprisingly, some concern was expressed about the state of her immune system. Skin tests were interesting, to say the least. She was highly sensitive to house dust mites and grass pollen, moderately sensitive to several mould species (Aspergillus, Alternaria, Candida, etc.), and mildly reactive to dog. She then told me that her home was an environmental disaster area! They had problems with rising damp, and the wine cellar (they had a wine cellar!) was very damp and musty. As it happens, they were about to move house anyway, so they paid particular attention when looking at new property to avoid mouldy conditions. She improved dramatically within weeks of the move, and remains well at the time of writing (three years later). *Asthma can be triggered by mould allergy!*

Bartley is an accountant who loves to forget about it all on horseback in an open field. So he was particularly upset to realise that he was starting to wheeze every time he went near his horse. He was perfectly well at other times. Skin tests confirmed his allergy: within ten minutes of scratching his arm with horse allergen he produced an enormous response. He was not allergic to anything else. Horse allergen is a potent one, and it is capable of triggering a severe and rapidly progressive asthmatic attack. *Asthma can be triggered by animals!*

John Hamilton was Archbishop of St Andrews in the sixteenth century. He had asthma. He also had a lot of money. Displeased with local treatment, he called for a renowned physician, Jerome Cardan of Pavia. Jerome travelled from Italy to Scotland with nothing much more than his bag. He took one look at the sorry priest puffing and wheezing in his bed. 'Get rid of that feather quilt!' he exclaimed, turned on his heel and returned to his lodgings. This may have been the shortest consultation in history, but the cleric's recovery was so complete that he rewarded the good doctor with 1,400 pieces of gold, and a gold chain for his neck. *Asthma can be triggered by an allergy to feathers!*

2. A few examples of asthma triggered by foods

Kevin was a four-year-old boy plagued with allergies. Mum and Dad knew that he was allergic to eggs. They made him extremely ill. Within ten minutes of eating them he would break out in a rash of hives and vomit violently. He also had eczema, asthma and rhinitis. Finally, and this is the reason his parents brought him to the Allergy Clinic, he had become hyperactive in recent months. 'He was always an active child,' they said. 'But this is ridiculous! He gets mood swings, loses his temper, and disrupts his Montessori class.' We put him on the Low Allergy Diet in the hope of improving his mood and behaviour. He enjoyed great relief from all his symptoms within ten days of his diet. 'His mood is much lighter, and he is now so pleasant,' his parents told me. 'Not only that, but his asthma, eczema and rhinitis are better than they have been for years.' *Asthma can be triggered by allergy to food — particularly when other symptoms of food allergy are present!*

Bernard was a little older than Kevin when I first met him. He also had a long history of asthma, and he too had other symptoms of food allergy. In particular, he frequently complained of bellyache and headache. Every day, he took two inhalers and one tablet to control his asthma. Notwithstanding his medication, he had a constant cough. In addition, he had several bad attacks each year requiring treatment with steroids. We put him on a ten-day Low Allergy Diet. By day seven, his lung function had improved quite dramatically. We then set about expanding his diet again, and managed to reintroduce all major food items without incident — until we came to soft drinks. Within thirty minutes of drinking a well-known branded lemon drink he developed an acute asthmatic attack. The drink was laden with metabisulphite — a preservative, and a recognised problem for some asthmatics. *Asthma can be triggered by an allergy to food additives!*

3. An example of asthma triggered by something at work
Let me remind you of Michael, the horticulturist we met in chapter 1. He had developed an allergy to lettuce — an allergen he met every day at work. He had occupational asthma. This subject is dealt with fully in chapter 8, so I won't go into it here. However, if you have asthma, remember that *asthma can be triggered by something at work!*

Asthma — the non-allergic triggers
We have already seen that asthma is characterised by hyper-reactive airways, and that they are very sensitive to change. This includes all manner of change, and not just the presence or absence of allergen. The non-allergic triggers include the following:

1. *Exercise* will spark off symptoms in almost all asthmatic patients. For some, this may be their only trigger. We call it exercise-induced asthma. These patients, like all asthmatics, have chronic inflammation of their airways, but they get symptoms only when they exert themselves.
2. *Changes in temperature* are a fairly common non-allergic trigger for asthma, especially noticeable when you go from a nice warm house to the cold air outdoors. The bronchial tubes don't like being hit by a cold draught and go into spasm.
3. *Emotion.* It is hard to imagine that asthma has ever conferred benefits on those who suffer it. But there is, at least, one great advantage which asthmatics had in the days of the Roman empire — they were exempt from torture! Soldiers knew that stress could bring on an attack, and the victim would be unable to talk. Apart from this isolated reprieve, asthma has no benefits for its victims. Present-day sufferers know all too well that the 'torture' of some of life's stresses, although less gruesome than the chamber, can aggravate their condition. That's not to say that asthma is 'all in the mind' — it's not. It's a disease of airway inflammation. If the airways were not inflamed, the asthmatic could be tortured like anyone else and not go into an asthmatic attack.

4. *Infections* can also trigger asthma. They do so in two ways. Firstly, the inflammatory response to the infecting bug compounds the underlying inflammation in the asthmatic airways. Secondly, the immune system sometimes becomes allergic to viral particles.

5. *Indigestion.* Gastro-oesophageal reflux is yet another trigger. This is when the junction between your gullet (oesophagus) and stomach (gastro-) is lax, which means that the acidic contents of the stomach can rush back into the gullet and irritate the bronchial tubes. Make sure to treat your indigestion if you have asthma!

6. *Hormones.* Finally, many women report that their asthma is more difficult to control in the premenstrual time. Indeed, more women than men are admitted to hospital with acute asthma, and many of these admissions occur just before or during the period (when levels of oestrogen are at their lowest). Conversely, and if you're lucky, your asthma could improve during pregnancy.

Are there any complications?

Complications arise in several settings:

1. the unrecognised or inadequately treated asthmatic
2. the patient who gets severe asthmatic attacks
3. patients with 'brittle' asthma (which is extremely difficult to control)

Unrecognised or inadequately treated asthmatics may suffer from sleep disruption, impaired concentration, fatigue and a general reduction in quality of life. Thankfully, in these days of greater awareness and better medicines, the rare complications of chest deformity and growth retardation are seldom seen. Adults with asthma may also suffer from fatigue, and in some cases this may be their only complaint.

Severe exacerbations of asthma are dramatic and alarming. The patient is, after all, unable to breathe! They may become so breathless that they cannot speak or pause for a drink. They adopt a classical forward-leaning stance to recruit more muscle for breathing. As the attack worsens they turn a shade of blue. They are now, of course, in urgent need of medical care. If such attacks are not treated, or do not respond to treatment, there is a risk of death.

Brittle asthma is very rare. It is a condition characterised by very frequent and very severe attacks.

Asthma and death

Before we go any further, let me make a few points about asthma and death. Yes, it happens, people do die from asthma, but we must not lose sight of the fact that such deaths are rare. Nevertheless, we must continually strive to reduce asthma mortality. Patients should always seek medical help if they are not getting relief from their usual asthma medication, even — and perhaps especially — if this happens in the middle of the night. *The most serious asthmatic attacks can be successfully handled if the patient comes forward in time.*

Asthmatics have an increased risk of death if . . .

1. they do not take their medication
2. their asthma is severe and difficult to control, even with medication
3. they do not have access to adequate medical treatment
4. they do not come forward in time for treatment during an attack

Bear in mind that asthma is extremely common. Indeed, it is the most common chronic disease of childhood. It is also a disease with a very wide spectrum of severity, ranging from the trivial to the life-threatening. For example, 11 per cent of the 1984 US Olympic team had asthma, and it did not interfere with performance! Similarly, many other famous sporting champions on this side of the Atlantic carry an inhaler. So, if you have asthma you should strive to lead a normal life. The vast majority of asthmatics do so. There is no need for patients or their parents to be in daily fear of their lives.

What can we do about asthma?

In treating asthma you will want to:

1. Identify your relevant allergens and reduce your exposure to them.
2. Identify your non-allergic triggers.
3. Reduce airway inflammation with medication.
4. Treat complications if and when they occur, without delay.
5. Consider a course of desensitisation to switch off allergies (my preferred option).

Check out the allergies!

The most helpful investigation for the patient with asthma is a detailed clinical history together with physical examination of the chest and a series of skin-prick tests (see chapter 17). This will give very reliable information on allergy to airborne allergens. Allergens commonly tested by skin-prick test include house dust mite, pollens, moulds and animal danders. Once you know which allergens are causing trouble you can take measures to reduce your exposure to them. The most common airborne culprit is, once again, the house dust mite. If you are allergic to this allergen you would be well advised to follow the avoidance measures detailed in appendix 1. Patients who have asthma and who have no positive skin-prick tests may wish to consider a Low Allergy Diet. Asthmatics should also strive to understand their non-allergic triggers.

Medical treatment for asthma

There are many different sets of guidelines for the treatment of asthma. I take mine from the *Global Initiative for Asthma*, a collaborative report published by the National Institutes of Health (USA) and the World Health Organization. The aim of treatment is to control the asthma, and that means (i) minimal or no symptoms, (ii) minimal or no need for medication, (iii) no need for emergency treatment, and (iv) no restriction on activities, including exercise. As a 'next best' option, medication may need to be taken on a daily basis to achieve control. If this is the case, a further aim of treatment is to minimise the side effects. We have some very useful drugs available to us, both in aerosol form for inhalation, and in tablet (or syrup) form for swallowing.

Inhalers

To put it simply, there are two categories of inhaler: one which relieves symptoms when they occur, the other which prevents them from occurring in the first place. We call these 'relievers' and 'controllers' respectively. If you go back for a minute to the underlying problem in the asthmatic chest, you will see that these medicines make a lot of sense. The reliever reduces spasm in the bronchial muscle. This immediately dilates (opens) the airway and allows easy breathing. Relievers are called bronchodilators. Controllers, on the other hand, are anti-inflammatory drugs. They seek to suppress the chronic inflammation of asthma, so reducing bronchial hyper-reactivity and the likelihood of asthma symptoms developing. Inhalers can be tricky little devices to get the hang of. Be sure to check your inhaler technique with your doctor, asthma nurse or pharmacist. Infants

and young children will need to use spacer devices (or a nebu-
liser) to ensure that the medicines end up in their chest!

Oral medicines

Tablets and syrups used in the treatment of asthma are also
divided into two broad categories: bronchodilators and anti-
inflammatories. Sometimes a drug will possess both qualities and
thus proves very useful in treating the more difficult cases.

Choosing medication

In deciding which medication to use, your doctor will categorise
your asthma by severity and treat accordingly. We have four
grades of severity, each with its own recommended treatment.
These are summarised as follows, but please discuss doses etc.
with your own doctor.

1. Intermittent Asthma
   Defined as:
   - Symptoms occur less than once per week, with brief
     exacerbations, and hardly any night-time trouble.
   Treated with:
   - Reliever: inhaler of short-acting bronchodilator as and
     when required, but should be less than once per day
   - Controller: none required

2. Mild Persistent Asthma
   Defined as:
   - Symptoms occur more than once per week, but not every
     day, with some limitation on exercise and some disrup-
     tion of sleep (less than twice a month).
   Treated with:
   - Reliever: inhaler of short-acting bronchodilator as and
     when required, but not more than four times a day
   - Controller: anti-inflammatory, by inhalation or orally, to
     be taken every day. Choose from steroid, cromoglycate or
     nedocromil inhalers; or a theophylline oral preparation.

3. Moderate Persistent Asthma
   Defined as:
   - Symptoms occur every day. They affect activity and sleep,
     with night-time symptoms occurring more than once a
     week.
   Treated with:
   - Reliever: inhaler of short-acting bronchodilator as and
     when required, but not more than four times a day

- Controllers: inhaler of anti-inflammatory steroid and long-acting bronchodilator (inhaled or swallowed) to be taken every day

4. Severe Persistent Asthma
Defined as:
- Symptoms are continuous. There are frequent exacerbations. Night-time symptoms are also frequent and activities are limited by symptoms.

Treated with:
- Reliever: inhaler of short-acting bronchodilator as and when required, even if it means more than four times a day
- Controllers: inhaler of anti-inflammatory steroid and long-acting bronchodilator (inhaled or swallowed) to be taken every day. May need to take steroids orally and continuously as well.

The *Global Initiative for Asthma* also stresses, at each and every point, the importance of avoiding or controlling your triggers, be they allergic or non-allergic. Thus, if you have intermittent asthma, and you start using your short-acting bronchodilator more than once a week, you will need to review your triggers before/as you upgrade your treatment to the next step on the scale. This holds true for all grades of asthma, and I repeat without embarrassment: if you begin to lose control, review your triggers.

Could it be anything else?

Yes! Other conditions may mimic asthma, in that they present with shortness of breath, cough or wheeze. The diagnostic feature of true asthma is *reversible* airflow limitation. Your doctor can demonstrate this quite simply. In adults, we must differentiate between asthma and . . .

- chronic bronchitis and emphysema, but the airflow limitation here is *irreversible.* In other words, they will not be helped by asthma medication. It is possible, of course, to have a mixed disease, with some asthma and some bronchitis.
- heart disease, which may present with shortness of breath and a wheeze
- rhinitis or chronic sinusitis, which give a post-nasal drip and chronic cough
- allergic lung diseases, such as farmer's lung, bird fancier's

lung, etc. These are allergic diseases which result from exposure to occupational or hobby-related allergens.

- panic attacks
- something else entirely!

Mandy is a busy mother of three, and she has a cough that just won't go away. It all started four months ago with a runny nose. In fact, Mandy thought it was a simple 'cold', but it went down to her chest a few days later, and stayed there ever since. She was bringing up white phlegm. Her doctor gave her several courses of antibiotic, but symptoms persisted and the question of asthma was now raised. Going into the story in a little more detail it transpired that Mandy's cough was quite characteristic. It occurred in spasms. When it did occur she coughed and coughed until her chest hurt. Sometimes she coughed so deeply that she vomited. However, these episodes were getting less frequent and less severe as the months went by. Mandy had whooping cough!

In young children, we must remember that:

- Wheeze is *not* synonymous with asthma.
- Recurrent viral infection is sometimes the only cause of recurrent wheeze.
- Something 'going down the wrong way' may cause a wheeze, such as recurrent milk inhalation.

6   *Allergy and the Eyes: Allergic Conjunctivitis and Related Disorders*

Healthy eyes

Have a look at yourself in the mirror. You will see, in each eye . . .

- the pupil, a small black spot in the centre of the eye. It dilates in the shade and constricts in the light.
- the iris, a circular structure around the pupil which gives us the colour of our eyes
- the cornea, a transparent dome-shaped structure which covers the iris and pupil
- the sclera, or the 'white' of the eye
- the conjunctiva, a very delicate lining on the inside of the eyelid and on the white of the eye. There is no conjunctival membrane over the cornea.
- the eyelid margin, from which the eyelashes emerge
- the eyelids themselves, which cover the eye when closed
- the periorbital skin, which includes the lids and extends from the eyebrows above to the cheekbone below, like the eye patches on a Panda bear!

In health, the eyelids serve to protect, lubricate and cleanse the eye, and particularly the cornea. Allergic disease affects only the external eye, from the conjunctiva outwards, i.e. the conjunctiva, the eyelids and the periorbital skin. The eyelids are very delicate, being only 0.55 mm thick. This explains why it is so vulnerable to contact allergy and irritation. However, the most common eye disorder by far is allergic conjunctivitis.

CASE HISTORY

Jim was a fourteen-year-old boy whose mother brought him to the clinic because he was always blinking. All day, every day. He had also taken to rubbing his eyes. They were itchy, and this was his only way of obtaining relief. However, rubbing his eyes only made them worse in the long run. The day I saw him, he had the appearance of someone struggling with a hangover! His eyes were bleary, red and tired-looking. He also admitted to symptoms of rhinitis, namely bouts of sneezing and a runny nose. Interestingly, he knew that all symptoms got worse when he visited his granny — she had three cats. He was prescribed an anti-allergy eye drop. This gave him complete relief within days of starting treatment. His response was so complete that no further action had to be taken with his allergies (although he still had to be careful with the cats). Jim had allergic conjunctivitis.

What is allergic conjunctivitis?

Allergic conjunctivitis is an inflammatory disorder of the delicate lining of the inner aspects of the eyelids. As in other allergic disorders, there is a full-blown inflammatory reaction raging within the conjunctiva. Symptoms will occur whenever there is contact with a relevant allergen, and will subside when the allergen is no longer present. The symptoms include:

1. itchy eyes, *always* — although this may feel more like a burning sensation.
2. watering eyes, with tears sometimes pouring out of the eyes.
3. swollen and painful eyelids
4. bloodshot eyes

Allergic conjunctivitis always affects both eyes simultaneously — unless one eye has been 'contaminated' with an allergen. For example, a patient who is allergic to dog hair and strokes a dog, then innocently rubs one eye with the same hand could experience a bout of conjunctivitis in that eye. Similarly, allergic conjunctivitis hardly ever occurs in isolation; it is nearly always associated with allergic rhinitis. Think about it. Any (airborne) allergen which gets into your eye will also get up your nose! A diagnosis of allergic conjunctivitis should be critically re-examined if there is no rhinitis present.

Who gets it?

Anybody can, but it's much more common in patients with a history of other allergic disease. It occurs more commonly in males of all ages.

Will they grow out of it?

Allergic conjunctivitis is usually a long-term disorder, with very little by way of spontaneous remission. Notwithstanding, if you can identify and remove the cause of your symptoms you stand a great chance of obtaining relief. Read on!

What causes it?

Allergic conjunctivitis is most commonly caused by an allergic reaction to something in the air. Symptoms will come and go with the allergen. Thus, if your allergen is a seasonal one, your symptoms will be seasonal. If, on the other hand, your allergen is constantly present (perennial), so will your symptoms be.

Allergic triggers of conjunctivitis

The allergic triggers are numerous and include:

1. inhalant allergens
   * pollen: grass, tree and weed
   * house dust mites
   * mould spores
   * animal danders and feathers
2. ingested allergens
   * food
3. contact allergens
   * cosmetics
   * contact lenses, and their
   * cleansing solutions
4. occupational allergens
   * see chapter 8

1. Inhalant allergens may cause perennial conjunctivitis

Vincent had made a name for himself locally by winning every tennis competition in his age group. He was still at school, but hoped to get a tennis scholarship abroad in a couple of years. Things were looking up, as they say. And they were, except for one thing: he had allergy problems — asthma, rhinitis and conjunctivitis, to be exact. He wheezed and coughed every day. He also ran out of breath before he should have done, and his tennis was beginning to falter as a result. The 'bunged-up nose' he could live with; the nickname of 'Sneezy' he could live with; even the asthma he could live with; but the eyes — that was another story. They were red. They were extremely itchy, and they watered constantly. Symptoms were most severe at night in bed, but they were also troublesome during the day. There was just no let-up. Day after day, after week, after month, for the past three years, and getting worse. He had also developed a corneal deformity (keratoconus) and was in need of a corneal graft. Skin tests confirmed the allergic nature of his problem: he was highly sensitive to grass, weed, tree, dust mites, house dust, animal danders and feathers. His exposure to these allergens was perennial. So were his symptoms. A course of desensitisation brought about a rapid and significant improvement in all of his allergies.

Inhalant allergens may cause seasonal conjunctivitis

This is perhaps the most common of all eye complaints: the seasonal conjunctivitis which is part and parcel of hay fever. Indeed, sometimes it is the most prominent symptom of hay fever. (See p. 55). Young Eileen is a case in point. She is now aged seven years and has had hay fever for the past three summers. 'Well actually,' her mother said, 'summer starts very early for Eileen, she sometimes sneezes in March!' Interestingly, her first symptom turns out to be a rash 'like a nettle burn' on the arms. She then starts to sneeze, and finally the eyes become red, swollen and itchy. The rash and the nasal symptoms are trivial compared to the eye symptoms. Skin tests confirm the clinical suspicion of silver birch and grass pollen allergy. This explains her 'early summer' and the persistence of symptoms throughout the grass pollen season (May–August). Eileen had no allergic symptoms throughout the rest of the year.

Inhalant allergens may cause situational conjunctivitis

Fergal remembers having eczema as a young lad, but this seldom affects him these days, apart from the occasional flare-up on his hands. What was bothering him now was the fact that he had to stop his horse-riding lessons. Every time he goes to the stables he gets a runny nose and watery eyes. Symptoms persist for as long as he insists on staying near horses, and subside completely within a few hours of leaving them. He has no symptoms if he stays away from his allergen. Skin tests confirmed his allergy, and further revealed potential problems with house dust mites and grass pollen. That's when he remembered his childhood asthma. He'd grown out of it, but he remembers that it was always worse when he was made to clean his bedroom.

2. Ingested allergens may cause conjunctivitis

Food allergy can cause conjunctivitis, but never in isolation. There will always be other symptoms of generalised food allergy, and these are usually much more serious than the conjunctivitis. Consequently, they will attract far more attention to themselves, and rightly so. The conjunctivitis becomes almost a non-event in medical terms.

The eyes are frequently affected by angioedema, a condition characterised by swelling of the eyelids. This may be so severe that the patient is unable to open their eyes until the swelling subsides.

3. Contact conjunctivitis

Don't forget about the things we touch, the contact allergies we discussed in chapter 3.II. As was the case with contact dermatitis, contact conjunctivitis may be allergic or irritant. It may also be associated with eyelid or periorbital dermatitis. Women are more at risk simply because they use more make-up. Here are some of the culprits.

- Cosmetics
  Applied to the eyelids, they may cause stinging and burning of the eyes during — or shortly after — application. This is usually transitory, with no objective evidence of irritation (the eye doesn't necessarily look red). It happens when irritant chemicals evaporate from the product (alcohol, isoparaffins, propylene glycol, sunscreen, soaps). Continued use may result in tolerance.
- Mascara
  Water-based mascara contains soap emulsifiers which may be irritating. Patients affected should use anhydrous or cake mascara.
  Mascara may accumulate under the conjunctiva and cause a more permanent irritation.
- Eyeshadow
  Some of these can be irritating. Try different kinds until you find one that suits you.

- Preservatives
  Especially parabens, which are found in virtually all eye cosmetics.
- Hair dyes
  Paraphenylenediamine and ammonium persulphate (platinum blonde) may induce dermatitis of the eyelids without affecting the scalp.
- Contact lens solutions
  Some preservatives in ophthalmic preparations may induce conjunctivitis and lid dermatitis.
- False eyelashes
  The adhesive may contain rubber latex, cellulose gums, casein-alkali or other resin.
- Eyelash curlers
  These can cause nickel dermatitis of the eyelids in nickel-sensitive subjects.
- Tissues
  These may be treated with perfume, formaldehyde or benzylkonium chloride — all of which may irritate or cause an allergy.
- Matches
  The relevant allergen here may become airborne! Being near a match-user is enough to induce eyelid dermatitis in sensitive subjects.
- Newsprint and carbon paper
  These may be irritating to the eyes.
- Other irritants include:
  household sprays, insecticides, animal hairs and occupational volatile chemicals

An example of contact allergic conjunctivitis

Mrs Neary was a middle-aged woman used to a good social life. As such, she had frequent cause to 'make herself up', and very glamorous she was too! She knew that cheap jewellery gave her a rash, but that didn't bother her because she didn't like cheap jewellery anyway. She was bothered by a recurrent rash on her eyelids, though. She couldn't understand it, having never suffered from the like before. Patch tests confirmed her sensitivity to nickel, but they also revealed a problem with one of her favourite moisturisers. It contained avocado, and she had become allergic to it. 'But I've used it for years!' she protested. (You've heard it all before, right?) She had sensitised herself to it

over time. 'But why are my hands not affected then?' she persisted. 'Because the skin over your eyes is only 0.55 mm thick,
and it's very delicate, that's why!' All she had to do now was
avoid the offending allergen. She should also be careful not to
handle nickel (coins, keys, cutlery, etc.) as this could contribute
to periorbital dermatitis as well.

The outcome is not always so clear for patients with suspected cosmetic allergy. Some unfortunates have 'status cosmeti-
cus' — a non-specific irritation to virtually all cosmetics. To
confound matters, they may have no outward sign of irritation
or allergy, but they complain of burning or stinging whenever
they wear cosmetics. Some of them will have slight redness over
the cheeks, with or without slight swelling of the eyelids, but
nothing more substantial than this. Treatment? Avoid all cosmetics!

Non-allergic triggers of conjunctivitis

In common with other allergic diseases (such as eczema, rhinitis
and asthma), allergic conjunctivitis may be aggravated by non-
allergic triggers. Failure to understand this could lead to many a
wild-goose chase. Maureen was one such patient. She had
moved into the area some three years earlier, and since doing so
developed 'hay fever' symptoms. Her most troublesome symptom was watering of the eyes, but she also had rhinitis. Her
symptoms were particularly bad whenever she went outdoors
during the summer months. She was convinced that something
in the air was affecting her. However, the skin tests failed to
show a relevant summer allergy. She was not allergic to any of
the pollens. Nor was she allergic to mould. Her only positive
reaction was to our old friend, the house dust mite. This didn't
fit with her expectations, and she remained convinced that 'we
were missing something'. Going back into her history, she told
me that her eyes were especially bad on bright, windy days.
'Maybe it's the silage, or the fertiliser being spread by neigh-
bouring farmers,' she thought out loud, 'They never did that
near my last house, you know.' Maureen had an allergic conjunctivitis and rhinitis related to the house dust mite. Her 'seasonal exacerbations' were in fact the result of non-allergic
triggers: the combination of wind and sunlight. Other non-
allergic triggers include inert dusts, such as chalkdust and the
chemical vapours commonly found in household products.

Are there any complications?

Allergic conjunctivitis is a miserable condition. It can disrupt academic performance and summer holidays, and impair the overall quality of life. It can be particularly nasty when associated with eczema, because it may affect the cornea, the transparent part of the eye through which we see the outside world. Allergic inflammation of the cornea can result in scarring, ulceration, cataract formation and corneal deformity. We call this 'atopic keratoconjunctivitis': *atopic* referring to the allergic disposition, and *kerato-* referring to the corneal involvement.

Atopic keratoconjunctivitis

Dermot was a fifteen-year-old schoolboy with several years of itchy, watering eyes. He also had a history of rhinitis and asthma. His eyes remained itchy in spite of anti-allergy eye drops and antihistamine tablets. His only relief came about by vigorously rubbing the eyes. His action was quite classical: he would press his curled index finger over his closed eye, and rub in a circular motion. And I mean rub! The eye surgeon diagnosed atopic keratoconjunctivitis with corneal deformity. His cornea had lost its nice smooth dome-shaped appearance, and looked more like the oval end of a rugby ball! We call this conical deformity 'keratoconus'. Dermot now needed a corneal graft (and here's one more good reason to sign your donor card!); without a healthy cornea from a donor eye, he would go blind. But how would a graft survive all this rubbing? The eye surgeon referred him to the Allergy Clinic for help with the allergic aspects of his disease. From the history, we suspected that certain airborne allergens were making him worse: house dust, animal danders, feathers and grass pollen all made his eyes intensely itchy. He also noticed that perfumes, and the like, could aggravate his symptoms. Having confirmed his allergies by skin tests, we started him on a course of desensitisation. He has had four injections over the past eight months and his symptoms are much better controlled. Specifically, the itch and the rubbing have ceased, and the surgeon is now ready to proceed with the graft.

What can we do about allergic conjunctivitis?

In treating allergic conjunctivitis you will want to:

1. Identify your relevant allergens and reduce your exposure to them.

2. Understand your non-allergic triggers.
3. Reduce conjunctival inflammation with medication.
4. Consider a course of desensitisation to switch off your allergies.

Skin-prick and patch tests will go a long towards identifying your allergies. There is no place for dietary investigation in this disorder. Once you know which allergens are causing your trouble you will be better placed to avoid them. Desensitisation is an effective therapeutic option. Meanwhile, we have several medical preparations which effectively reduce symptoms. These can be applied directly into the eye.

- Antihistamine eye drops
  These are quite safe and give rapid relief. They should be taken as long as symptoms persist. That means that 'hay fever' patients with seasonal allergic conjunctivitis need to take them throughout the pollen season. Perennial conjunctivitis requires continuous treatment. Antihistamines may also be taken orally.
- Corticosteroid eye drops
  These are very powerful, but should be used only under the close supervision of a doctor.
- Bear in mind that you could be allergic to a preservative or other ingredient of the eye treatment — another case of allergy treatment causing allergy!

Could it be anything else?

Yes! Allergic conjunctivitis should not be confused with:

- Vernal keratoconjunctivitis
  Vernal conjunctivitis occurs in allergic individuals, but it is not necessarily an allergy! It occurs most commonly in young boys during the spring and summer months (*vernal* referring to *spring*). Having said that, it can occur in girls and it can be perennial. The fact that many of these patients also have positive skin tests may confuse matters further. This simply means that allergic children are more likely to get vernal conjunctivitis, not that the condition is, in itself, an allergic one. If in doubt, check out the nose! If there are no symptoms of allergic rhinitis, then the conjunctivitis is not allergic (rule of thumb). The symptoms of vernal conjunctivitis are very similar to the allergic ones, namely itch, watering and redness of the eyes. In addition, there may be a thick white 'stringy'

discharge from the eye — a result of prolonged inflammation. The good news is this: most patients will grow out of their vernal conjunctivitis with the advent of puberty. For this reason I think of *vernal* in terms of the spring of life, rather than the spring of the *seasons*!

- Giant papillary conjunctivitis
  We do come up with some great names, don't we? This one applies to an inflammatory response to contact lenses, be they hard or soft, but more commonly soft. Patients complain of itch, watering eyes and discomfort when wearing their lenses. Vision may also be impaired, and the lens may move about excessively. Treatment options include (i) wearing glasses, (ii) wearing disposable lenses, (iii) adopting scrupulous lens hygiene measures, with or without a prescribed anti-inflammatory eye drop.

- Infective conjunctivitis

- Bacterial infections of the conjunctiva, and particularly of the eyelid margins, are not uncommon. Blepharitis is the name given to the latter. Viral (and other) infections may also occur.

- Seborrhoeic blepharo-conjunctivitis
  Sometimes the eyelids become inflamed as part of another skin disease called seborrhoeic dermatitis. In this case, there will be other patches of dermatitis in the eyebrows and scalp. Blepharitis will always cause a bit of conjunctivitis, hence the amazing name!

- Dry eyes (keratoconjunctivitis sicca)
  Frequently confused with allergic conjunctivitis, this condition primarily affects women of menopausal age, but it may also affect men. It is commonly found in patients with arthritis.

In all of these cases, itch is *not* a prominent feature. Rather, patients complain of irritation, or a burning sensation in the eyes. They may feel 'gritty'. Treatment depends on the cause, so it is important to get the diagnosis right.

7   *Allergy and the Mouth*

The healthy mouth

Have another look in the mirror. This time examine your mouth, and notice . . .

- the oral mucosa — the smooth pink lining inside the cheeks and lips
- the palate — the roof of the mouth — hard towards the front, and soft towards the back. That thing dangling down in the middle is called the uvula.
- the gums — or gingiva, out of which the teeth emerge
- the throat — or oropharynx, everything further back than the tongue
- the glottis — shaped like a small shoehorn, peeping up at you from deep in the throat (you may have difficulty seeing it!)
- the tongue — with numerous taste buds of variable size, smaller towards the front, larger towards the back
- the salivary glands — Point your tongue towards the roof of your mouth. Do you notice two worm-like structures sitting under the tongue? There is one on each side, converging towards the midline. These are the sublingual salivary glands. There are other salivary glands flowing into the mouth, but they are not so readily visible.

- the lips   smooth and pink, with a clear margin where the mucosal surface meets the skin
- the perioral skin   the area of skin around the outside of the mouth, extending from the nose above to the chin below

You will notice that space is limited in the mouth, and particularly at the back of the throat. Food and air have to share this space, so we rely on the glottis to control the traffic. It stays open during breathing (to allow air into the lungs), and shuts down during a swallow (to prohibit food from entering the windpipe).

1. ORAL ALLERGY SYNDROME
CASE HISTORY

It all started two years ago for Caroline. She was eleven years old when she first noticed that something was amiss. Her mouth went numb and her upper lip swelled after eating melon. It passed of its own accord, she shrugged her shoulders and forgot about it. Two months later she had a similar experience, this time with an apple. Her lips and tongue felt 'funny', a bit numb, or maybe there was a slight tingle (she found it hard to describe). Within weeks, she was reacting in this way to carrots, peppers, lettuce, kiwi and cherries. By the time I saw her, she had stopped eating *all* fruit and vegetables. However, she discovered that *if these foods were cooked* first they caused her no trouble — except, perhaps, for carrot. Of some concern was the fact that she was now likely to get chest pain and shortness of breath if she inadvertently ate a forbidden food, such as when she visited a friend and the vegetables were cooked al dente (slightly raw, the way they should be). She denied any other allergic history, and this is the only unusual aspect of her case. On skin-testing she reacted *as expected* to silver birch pollen (see below). She also had positive skin tests to egg, potato, peanut, soy bean, orange, strawberry, pear, banana, lemon, coconut, grape, peas, tomato and onion! I gave up testing her at that stage, and I did a blood test to confirm that the skin tests were truly positive, and not just a quirk of her funny skin, or my imagination! Every single blood test came back positive. On blood test, she was allergic to all of the foods mentioned above, but she was also positive to grass pollen and mould! Caroline had a classical case of Oral Allergy Syndrome.

What is Oral Allergy Syndrome?

Oral Allergy Syndrome (OAS) is an acute allergic reaction to diverse vegetables and fruit. Symptoms occur upon contact with the offending food and are usually restricted to the mouth and throat, the areas of contact. In this sense, OAS is a form of contact urticaria and angioedema (see p. 42). However, if the patient fails to heed the allergic warning and swallows the food, other symptoms may develop: the patient may vomit, have diarrhoea, break out in a rash, become short of breath, or even collapse into a life-threatening shock (see chapter 9).

The condition starts with a (usually mild) reaction to one or two foods. The sensitivity then spreads to affect other foods, and this often occurs in recognised clusters. For example, some patients are allergic to hazelnut, apple, pear, potato and carrot; whilst others react to melon, watermelon and tomato; or to peach, apricot, plum, etc. These foods are clustered because they belong to the same families, and they all look alike to the immune system. For some patients the allergic sensitivity then spreads to a whole range of fruit and vegetables across the botanical divides.

Cooking a food changes the shape of its allergen(s) — in much the same way that burning your hair makes it shrivel and curl! The immune system does not recognise these denatured allergens, and does not react against them. The exception is carrot, whose allergen is particularly resistant to heat. This is the reason why many patients with this condition are able to tolerate the cooked version of their allergic foods. The characteristics of Oral Allergy Syndrome can be summarised as follows:

- a rapid onset of symptoms after contact with offending foods (less than thirty minutes):
  - itching or tingling of the lips, mouth and throat
  - blisters on the inside of the mouth
  - swelling of the lips, and/or tongue, and/or throat
- more serious symptoms may occur if the food is swallowed:
  - vomiting
  - diarrhoea
  - generalised urticaria
  - difficulty breathing
  - shock

Who gets it?

Oral Allergy Syndrome occurs almost exclusively in those who are allergic to pollen (but not all pollen-sensitive persons will get it). If you are allergic to grass or weed pollen, there is a 40 per cent chance that you will have symptoms after eating certain fruits or vegetables; and if you are allergic to silver birch pollen, there is a 60 per cent chance that you will have symptoms when you eat apples! If one accepts that 10 per cent of the general population is allergic to one pollen or another, we can assume that some 4 to 6 per cent will experience a degree of Oral Allergy Syndrome.

Will they grow out of it?

No.

What causes it?

Oral Allergy Syndrome is a syndrome of cross-reactions. That is, the immune system reacts across a range of allergens which, to it, all look alike. That's why it occurs mostly in those who are first allergic to plant pollens. The pollen allergen 'looks like' fruit and vegetable allergens. Hence, once a patient is sensitised to pollen, they can easily cross-react to fruits and vegetables. Another possible explanation is that many plants share the same allergens, not just ones that look alike. Profilin and a glycoprotein, which are present throughout the plant kingdom, are possible examples of this.

Are there any complications?

Apart from the great nuisance of having to be careful with raw or undercooked foods, Oral Allergy Syndrome patients are at risk of serious allergic reactions if they swallow their allergen raw. Some 10 per cent of these will experience swelling of the glottis — a swelling that could threaten the airway. A further 2 per cent will get a generalised life-threatening reaction (see chapter 9).

What can we do about it?

Patients must be very careful to eat only well-cooked fruits and vegetables. They must also bear in mind that, even then, some foods (such as carrot) will not be safe. An anti-allergy medicine called Nalcrom may also help to reduce symptoms (if taken thirty minutes before food). It works by stabilising mast cells in the gut. Anyone who has experienced a life-threatening reaction should read chapter 9. Finally, some patients will benefit from a course of desensitisation (see chapter 18).

Could it be anything else?

The clinical history of Oral Allergy Syndrome is usually very clear-cut, and suspicions can be confirmed by skin and blood tests. It is, of course, possible to get similar symptoms from allergy to other foods, such as fish or peanut, without having the full syndrome outlined above. Similarly, aspirin and related drugs may sometimes cause the same trouble.

Oral Allergy Syndrome should not be confused with:

- 'Pineapple mouth'
  A burning excoriation of the lips and perioral skin after eating pineapple — which contains an irritant enzyme.
- 'Citrus mouth'
  Similar to pineapple mouth, but this time a contact dermatitis caused by limonene, an oil found in the skin of citrus fruit, dill, caraway and celery.
- Non-allergic airway obstruction
  Judy and Anne had taken their elderly mother out for an afternoon at the fair. They were on their feet for hours, going from stall to stall, stopping only to chat with old friends. Towards evening they decided on a meal, took their seats in a restaurant and ordered from the menu. The chat continued apace as the food was served. Mother was in great form. But she suddenly gasped for air and stood up, petrified, with one hand holding her throat, the other stretched out for help. Her mouth was open wide in a desperate bid to catch a bigger breath. 'Take a drink, mum!' cried one of the girls, pouring out the water. But the poor woman couldn't pause long enough to lift the glass. They brought her down to the ladies' room, but she wouldn't go in. She was ashen-faced, weak-ened by the struggle, and afraid to be left alone. 'What on earth is wrong?' one daughter asked pleadingly, but she couldn't answer them. Then a man from a nearby table approached the woman as she steadied herself against the wall, still clutching her throat. 'What happened?' he asked, 'Did something go down the wrong way?' She nodded, her eyes communicating all at once her fright and her relief at being understood. He asked again, 'Are you choking on something?' She nodded again, yes. Pushing the daughters

aside, the stranger forced the terrified woman to lie face down on the floor. He stood over her body, one foot on each side, and stooped down to wrap his arms around her belly. Then he yanked her up between his legs and, just as suddenly, dropped her violently onto his firmly clasped hands. A lump of fish shot out of her mouth, and the woman took the biggest, noisiest, happiest breath of her life. She stood up, still trembling, and spoke her gratitude. When she looked at it, the lump of fish was really quite small. Nevertheless, it had nearly taken her life. There isn't much space in the throat!

A word about dental allergy

Susan is an eighteen-year-old student nurse. She was referred to the Allergy Clinic by her dentist because of a rather frightening reaction she had in the dental chair. She told me that one of her cheeks started to swell just as the dentist completed a filling. Her tongue was also swollen, so much so that her speech was slurred. The dentist packed her off to the hospital, where she was admitted for observation. Her blood pressure was low, her heart was racing and she felt a bit faint. She was put on a drip to support her blood pressure, and she was given an antihistamine injection to reduce the swelling. This treatment was quite successful, and she was discharged the following day with no ill effects. Susan had a reaction to dental material(s). We now had to find out what it was that caused her such grief, lest she suffer it again. There were several possibilities. She could have been allergic to the dentist's latex gloves, the local anaesthetic, the mouthwash, or indeed any other material used during her treatment. It was also possible that she had a non-allergic reaction to the local anaesthetic. Such reactions can cause swelling, low blood pressure, fast heartbeat and even fainting.

A word about oral infection

Patricia also thought that she was allergic to 'something used by the dentist'. The day after her last visit she developed a crop of mouth ulcers. Her mouth was also generally sore and a bit swollen. The ulcers healed spontaneously within nine days, and she had completely recovered by the time I saw her. Her clinical history was fully consistent with a diagnosis of herpes (viral) infection in the oral mucosa and gums. We call this acute gingivostomatitis. Nevertheless, she was nervous about future dental treatment, so we patch-tested her anyway. The results were negative, suggesting once again that she had experienced a non-allergic event.

2. CONTACT ALLERGIC STOMATITIS
CASE HISTORY

Anne Marie had her first set of dentures fitted by the dentist some eight months ago. Everything was going well until she developed a stinging sensation on her tongue. She also complained that her sense of taste was altered, and that her mouth was 'generally sore'. She removed her plate for a few days and her symptoms gradually settled. She then returned to the dentist, and was given a new plate in the hope that this would solve her problem. It didn't. All of her symptoms returned within a week. Inside her mouth, one could see only a mild redness together with a few blisters on her palate — where she had most contact with the dental plate. In spite of the paucity of visible disease, Anne Marie had a contact allergic stomatitis.

What is contact allergic stomatitis?

Contact allergic stomatitis is, to put it simply, a contact allergic 'dermatitis in the mouth' (stoma). There are, however, some important differences between the two conditions.

1. Stomatitis is less common than dermatitis because:
   - allergens are not in contact with the mouth for long
   - the saliva dilutes and washes away allergens
   - the lining of the mouth has a great blood supply so that absorbed allergens are quickly removed from the site of contact. There are two exceptions to this rule, namely cases caused by contact with dental appliances/materials and by chewing pencils, jewellery, etc.
2. The subjective symptoms of stomatitis are much more prominent than the physical signs. Thus, patients frequently complain of:
   - loss of taste
   - burning in the mouth
   - numbness
   - pain

But the doctor, on the other hand, may see:
   - very little to account for the symptoms
   or
   - a hardly noticeable redness

or
- an angrier redness

and/or
- a little swelling

and/or
- a disappearance of buds on the tongue

and/or
- mouth 'ulcers'

3. Contact allergic stomatitis is usually limited to areas of contact. Rash does not spread to adjacent areas in the mouth. Again, this is in contrast to allergic dermatitis, where rash may spread quite a distance from the site of contact. Having said that, allergic stomatitis is frequently associated with contact allergic disease on the lips. In this case, the lips become dry, they flake, and they split open (fissures). We call this contact allergic cheilitis.

Who gets it?

Anybody can.

Will they grow out of it?

No.

What causes it?

Contact allergic stomatitis and cheilitis may be caused by:

- toothpaste
- mouthwash
- topical medication
- appliances and materials used by dentists
- lipstick
- nail varnish (biting nails increases risk)
- nickel (sucking jewellery increases risk)
- foods
- other contact allergens (see chapter 3.II)

Are there any complications?

Nothing too serious.

So, what can we do about it?

The best we can do is identify the relevant allergen and avoid it. Patch-testing will offer the best chance of a reliable result.

Could it be anything else?

Contact allergic disease in and around the mouth should not be confused with:

- Recurrent mouth ulcers
  These are painful sores inside the mouth and lips which affect 10 per cent of the population. They may occur in ones and twos, or in larger crops. They may be small or large, and last anything from seven to twenty-one days before they heal spontaneously. Only 4 or 5 per cent of these are allergic in origin.
- Denture damage
  Ill-fitting dentures may damage the oral mucosa. They are also more likely to become infected with thrush (candida). Some unfortunate women are afflicted with a generalised denture intolerance. They complain of discomfort without any evidence of allergy or disease.
- Vitamin deficiency
  Vitamin deficiency can look like stomatitis!
- Burning Mouth Syndrome
  This condition is characterised by a sensation of burning, or other painful feelings, in the mouth, related to the nervous system. It is akin to neuralgia, and may be helped by the use of specific medication to reduce the conduction of pain along nerve fibres.
- Dry Mouth Syndrome
  Salivary output decreases with age. Consequently, some elderly patients are left with a 'dry mouth'. They may experience some of the symptoms of stomatitis.
- Something else entirely!
  Larry was a sales representative who had recently been promoted to regional management. He presented with a ten-month history of painful swollen lips. 'Every morning,' he told me, 'I have to remove a layer of dead "skin" from my lips.' He also complained of pain and tingling around his mouth. He had no other symptoms. I spent considerable time going into all of the possible 'contacts' he may have had, not forgetting his cutlery, toothbrush, pencil, favourite mug, work-related allergens, girlfriend's lipstick and perfume, etc. Patch tests were entirely normal. The Low Allergy Diet failed. Avoidance (just-in-case) measures were unhelpful. I then came back to a subject with which he was uncomfortable. 'I

have failed to identify an allergen,' I said, 'and I feel we should have another look at your lip-biting.' He was in the habit of twisting his pursed lips to one side of his face whilst chewing on them! He had, in that sense, an 'artefactual' (self-inflicted) cheilitis.

8　Allergy on the Job

The healthy workplace

Every worker is entitled to a safe and healthy workplace. However, this chapter deals, not with questions of 'Health and Safety', but with the common allergic problems that arise in the course of employment — even when reasonable steps are taken to ensure a healthy work environment. Here are a few examples of what I mean.

CASE HISTORIES

Victoria was a hairstylist in her second year of training. She had a long-standing problem with rhinitis and sinusitis which she 'had learned to live with'. However, she had recently developed a chronic cough and had to take time off work as a result. She noticed that her cough cleared completely at home and started up again the day she returned to work. Consequently, she was sent home again, and the cough stopped. Patch tests were performed using materials with which she had regular contact at work. Not only did she develop a positive reaction on skin test, but she experienced a return of her cough together with wheeze, and a flare-up in her rhinosinusitis. An interesting aspect of this case is that individual allergens did not cause a problem, it was only when two of these were mixed together that she developed a positive reaction (and symptoms to match). That's when she realised that it was precisely these two substances that caused most trouble: when they were being mixed she started to wheeze, even if the mixing was being done by someone else in the salon. She had developed an **occupational asthma**.

Betty had worked her way up from the factory floor to quality control supervisor since joining a large manufacturing company two years ago. During this time she also had less welcome developments in that her nose started streaming and sneezing. At first she thought it was a cold. Then she thought she was just getting a lot of colds. Then she realised that something was wrong! She kept a diary and discovered that symptoms came on during the evening of every working day. That is, they started only when she was at home after work. She had minimal symptoms during the weekends, and no symptoms whatever during holidays. There was a lot of soldering going on at work, and Betty would frequently help out with this when they were busy, as they invariably were. Betty had developed an **occupational rhinitis.**

Catherine worked in a bakery on a part-time basis to supplement the family income. She enjoyed the work until she developed dermatitis. At first she thought it had nothing to do with work, so we put her on the Low Allergy Diet. To her great relief the rash cleared within a week, only to return when she started eating wheat. Skin tests confirmed that she was allergic to wheat, so she stayed away from it. The problem was, her rash came back whenever she tried to work in the bakery. She was advised to wear gloves when handling flour but this only partially reduced the severity of her rash. She was still inhaling the flour (everybody who works in a bakery does) and the only symptom of inhalant flour allergy may be a rash on the hands. Catherine had developed an **occupational dermatitis.**

Colm was a nurse in charge of a busy accident department. He came to the Allergy Clinic because of what he thought was a fairly straightforward problem. He gets sick whenever he eats banana, and he just wanted 'to check it out'. Colm didn't realise it, of course, but he was telling me that he was allergic to latex! Let me explain. In the first place, latex and banana are cross-reacting allergens: if you're allergic to one, you're likely to become allergic to the other. Secondly, Colm was a nurse. As such, he was at risk of developing a latex allergy — after all, 5 to 17 per cent of medical, nursing and dental workers are allergic to latex. Blood tests confirmed that Colm had antibodies in his blood against both latex and banana. He now had to make some fairly big decisions because continued exposure to latex could make him even more sensitive. Colm had developed an **occupational anaphylaxis** (see chapter 9).

Deborah recently graduated from university with a science degree. She went straight from college to work in a pharmaceutical firm. Within four months of starting the job, she developed urticaria. Her rash flared up almost as soon as she entered her laboratory, settled down when she left work in the evenings, disappeared altogether at weekends, and flared up again first thing on Monday morning. She had contact with several potential culprits. Our job was to find out which one had given her an **occupational urticaria**.

What is an occupational allergy?

By definition, an occupational allergy is one which is caused by exposure to a substance in the workplace. The range of possible symptoms is quite broad and includes:

1. asthma
and/or
2. rhinitis and sinusitis
and/or
3. urticaria
and/or
4. conjunctivitis
and/or
5. contact allergic dermatitis
and/or
6. anaphylaxis (fatal or near-fatal allergy)

These conditions are fully discussed in their own right elsewhere in this book. What is of particular interest to us here is that *they may be caused by something at work*. Now the question is: what about *your* asthma, *your* rhinitis, or *your* whatever? Is it possible that something in *your* work environment is causing the trouble? The first clue is often, but not always, the pattern of symptoms. You will have noticed that, in all but one of our case studies, a clear relationship exists between symptoms and the work environment. In these cases there was a significant reduction of symptoms away from work and a return of symptoms with a return to work. This is generally the case, especially in the initial stages of an occupational allergy. You will have also noticed that the symptoms may be either immediate (as with

Deborah's urticaria) or delayed (as with Betty's rhinitis). To confuse matters further, some patients have both immediate and delayed symptoms. However, all of these patterns may be lost if the allergy is allowed to continue unchecked. These are important points to remember when reflecting on the pattern of your own symptoms.

Who gets it?

Atopic individuals (who have a history of eczema, asthma, rhinitis and/or urticaria) are at greater risk of developing certain types of occupational allergy. In particular, they are at risk of grain, flour and animal allergy. However, anybody can develop an occupational allergy, irrespective of their past history. The risk has more to do with what they are exposed to at work than with any allergic problems they have had in the past.

Cases of occupational asthma have now been traced to over 200 substances, and this list continues to grow. The situation for occupational rhinitis is similar, although less well documented. In general, if something can give you asthma, it can also give you rhinitis. Certain occupations carry a greater risk of sensitisation. Some of the more troublesome allergens (and affected professions) include:

Allergen source	Affected workers
Animals	Handlers, laboratories, veterinarians, etc.
Enzymes (bacillus subtilis, papain, etc.)	Pharmaceutical, laboratory workers
Plants (hops, tea, buckwheat, tobacco)	Brewery, food processors, manufacturers
Latex (gloves)	Doctors, dentists, nurses, etc.
Grain dusts and mites	Millers, dockers, hauliers, etc.
Food dusts (wheat and rye)	Bakers and millers
Foods (salmon, crab and prawn)	Food processors and handlers
Gum acacia and tragacanth	Gum manufacturers
Metal salts (nickel, cobalt, platinum, etc.)	Metal processors

Drugs (penicillin, tetracycline, others)	Laboratory, pharmaceutical staff
Di-isocyanates	Plastics, polyurethane, varnish, paints
Anhydrides	Plastics, epoxy resins, adhesives
Persulphate salts	Hairdressers
Ethylenediamine	Photographers
Wood dusts (oak, mahogany, etc.)	Carpenters
Colophony	Soldering, electronics industry
Dyes	Clothing industry
Ethanolamine	Spray-painters

Will they grow out of it?

Most cases of occupational allergy will resolve if the patient is removed from the work environment *early on in the course of their disease*, although it may take up to two years for symptoms to resolve fully. Those who develop occupational asthma, and who are subjected to continued exposure, run the risk of being left with permanent asthma, *even if they get out of the situation at a later date*. A similar problem exists for the older worker who develops occupational contact allergic dermatitis. For this reason, workers should be offered compensation and medical retirement if they can prove that their allergic disease is caused *directly* by exposure to an allergen at work. Obviously, this would allow them the financial security required to get out of a situation which will permanently damage their health.

What causes it?

We don't know why some people develop occupational allergy and others don't. Apart from the risk of atopy mentioned above, there seems to be no way of predicting who will be affected and who will not. There is no doubt, however, that certain allergens are extremely strong sensitisers: that is, they have great potential to induce allergic reactions. Platinum is one example of this, with positive skin tests showing up in 15 per cent of those who work with it. Similarly, colophony is thought to induce asthma in 30 per cent of those exposed to it.

Are there any complications?

In addition to the usual complications of the various diseases themselves, those who develop occupational allergy have to make some serious decisions about their future employment. This problem has cut many a career short, and has dropped many a fine worker into financial hardship.

What can we do about it?

The best we can do — and we *must* do it — is identify the relevant allergens. Every adult with rhinitis, asthma and dermatitis should be assessed for occupational (and hobby) sensitivity. This will involve a detailed clinical history together with appropriate skin-prick and patch tests.

Could it be anything else?

As with so many of the allergic conditions already discussed, the most important distinction to bear in mind is the difference between an *allergic* symptom and an *irritant* one. Thus, occupational allergies should not be confused with:

- Non-allergic occupational triggers of asthma and rhinitis
  Many substances encountered at work may cause problems for the patient with pre-existing asthma and/or rhinitis. These include irritant chemicals and fumes, such as:
  — sulphur dioxide (oil industry)
  — chlorine (swimming pools)
  — diesel and petrol fumes
  — cosmetics
  — and even physical (non-chemical) triggers such as the temperature change in 'cold air rooms' (e.g. laboratories, walk-in freezers and abattoirs)
- Non-allergic occupational triggers of dermatitis
  Many of us are challenged by innumerable irritants in the course of our employment. Those with a history of contact allergic dermatitis, or even a past history of eczema, will be at greater risk of irritating their (more delicate) skin following contact with irritants. Be aware of:
  — soaps and detergents
  — disinfectants
  — metal salts
  — solvents
  — chemicals

— oils
— plants
— polishes etc.

- Reactive Airways Dysfunctional Syndrome

  In contrast to occupational asthma, in which workers become allergic to *an allergen over time*, the Reactive Airways Dysfunctional Syndrome (RADS) refers to the sudden development of 'asthma' after a significant *single exposure to an irritant*. Such exposures are invariably accidental, and usually involve noxious gases or vapours. By definition, RADS patients . . .

  — have no history of asthma before the exposure
  — have a significant (high-concentration) single exposure to toxic fumes or vapours
  — develop symptoms within twenty-four hours of the exposure
  — and still have symptoms three months after the exposure

  The symptoms of RADS mimic the symptoms of true asthma, namely cough, wheeze and shortness of breath. Furthermore, now that their bronchial tubes have been so irritated, simple stimuli such as dust or perfume can make them cough and wheeze. They don't have true asthma, they have very twitchy bronchial tubes, and this hyper-reactivity may persist for many years.

- Sick Building Syndrome

  The Sick Building Syndrome was first accorded formal recognition by the World Health Organization in 1982. It refers to a 'higher than expected' incidence of characteristic symptoms amongst workers in a given building. A building is considered 'sick' if 30 per cent, or more, of its occupants complain of the following:

  — Irritation of the eyes, which may be described as dry or watery, itchy, burning or smarting. There may also be difficulty wearing contact lenses.
  — Irritation of the nose, which may be described as itchy, 'runny' or blocked. Nosebleeds may also occur.
  — Irritation of the throat, with dryness of the throat and difficulty swallowing.
  — Irritation of the skin, which may be described as 'dry' or 'itchy' — with or without a rash.
  — Other symptoms including headache, fatigue, irritability and poor concentration.

You will notice, once again, that the symptoms here are all *irritative* rather than *allergic*. In Sick Building Syndrome, it is the work environment which is 'sick' — not the occupants per se. To put it another way, if the building was a 'healthier' environment, the occupants would be healthier too. The symptoms usually result from a combination of several irritant factors in the workplace which have an adverse cumulative effect on the people working in it. For example, the office may be too hot and too dry, and the equipment in it may be giving off substantial amounts of irritative chemicals, such as formaldehyde.

Those who know tell us that one-third of all new or remodelled buildings are, to some degree, 'sick'. Quite apart from the health implications for the workforce, there are several very good reasons to optimise the workplace. This will reduce sickness absence to a minimum, improve the morale of staff, improve industrial relations and increase productivity. It will also reduce the amount of time spent dealing with the health complaints of staff, as well as the expense of replacing and/or retraining them.

The assessment of a 'suspected sick building' should include a full consideration of:

1. Physical factors
   — the layout and design of the building
   — the work space
   — the lighting
   — the window type
   — the heating/ventilation mechanisms
   — and the extent to which these are under the direct control of individual members of staff
2. Indoor air quality factors
   — levels of carbon dioxide and oxygen
   — levels of volatile organic compounds and other chemicals
   — levels of dust
   — temperature and humidity
   — air movement
3. Biological factors
   — the presence of micro-organisms and/or their toxins
4. Psychological factors
   Health complaints within a workforce may be driven or complicated by psychological factors. The psychosocial environment can be assessed by asking occupants to rate:
   — their level of job satisfaction

— how clearly they understand their role in the firm
— the presence or absence of role conflict between colleagues
— the amount of work-related tension they have to cope with
— the stress of their workload
— whether they get on well with other members of staff
— and whether they get on well with those in management

A word about chemically induced food intolerance

Nancy worked as a technical assistant in a chemical plant. One day, she smelt something funny coming from one of the vents. She didn't recognise the smell, no one else seemed bothered by it and no alarm sounded. She continued working. One by one the laboratory personnel became ill. They started to cough, one of them vomited, and several developed headaches. Meanwhile the smell was getting stronger. They put two and two together, realised that they were dealing with a chemical accident and left the premises smartly. Nancy was admitted to hospital, and discharged a few days later without treatment. That was last year, and Nancy has never been right since. In particular, she still had headaches, muscle pains and dizziness. She was also tired, and could not manage much outside of her routine work. On closer questioning, Nancy admitted to other symptoms, including bloating of the abdomen, bouts of diarrhoea and the occasional tummy cramp. She also complained of an increased sensitivity to chemical smells, such as bleach, polish, perfume, and the like. We put her on the Low Allergy Diet and *all of her symptoms disappeared* within twelve days. She was pain-free for the first time since the accident. One by one we reintroduced foods and identified which ones were causing her trouble and which were safe. She is now well into a course of desensitisation to allow her to eat a wide and nutritious diet without suffering the ill effects of food intolerance. Nancy had developed multiple food intolerance as a complication of chemical toxicity at work.

SECTION 3

Fatal and Near-Fatal Allergy

9 *Anaphylaxis*

The 8th of November 1994 is for ever etched in our minds. It was the end of another busy day as we sat around with our three children, eating what was left of the Hallowe'en nuts, and catching up with each other's news. Our eldest daughter, Aisling, was then aged five. She started to cough, and complained of a sore throat whilst eating. I looked in her mouth and, finding nothing amiss, clapped her reassuringly on the back as doctors sometimes do. She then went upstairs to brush her teeth in preparation for bed, still complaining of pain. Her protests on the stairs were put down to another attack of the 'Shirley Temples'! By the time she reached the bathroom, her face was peppered with enormous hives, and her tongue was swollen with angry lumps. I threw a blanket around her, lifted her into my arms and rushed downstairs to the car. I was headed for hospital. On the way, she started to wheeze, and then slumped to one side in the back seat. I shouted at her: 'Aisling! Stay with me now, baby, stay with me!' But she could hardly speak. She was weak, very weak. I drove like a lunatic, one eye on Aisling, the other on the road; hazard lights, headlights and horn flashing and sounding as I weaved my way dangerously in and out of traffic. I thought I would lose her. But I knew that if I could just get her there alive she would have a chance. Adrenaline, that's what she needed now, and nothing else would do. I ran into the emergency department, trembling; by now her eyes were swollen like balloons, her breathing was noisy and distressed, and hives were spreading to the rest of her body. I handed her over to the medical staff and prayed. Aisling was in the throes of **anaphylaxis.**

I would estimate that her symptoms began within three or four minutes of eating nuts, and that another five minutes had elapsed before we reached hospital. Her symptoms were dramatic, and they developed at a terrifying pace. This was, without doubt, a potentially life-threatening situation. To our great joy, Aisling pulled through. But, sadly, others like her have been less fortunate. Each year, some six to eight people die from this sort of allergy in the British Isles.

The blood tests came back a few weeks later. They confirmed a definite allergy to Brazil nut. The other nuts, including peanut, did not show up in the blood. However, the skin test to peanut was most certainly positive. Aisling, for her part, was unable to sleep for about a month. She had got an awful fright. There is no doubt, however, that she now fully understands her situation. 'Thank you, Lord Jesus, that I didn't die when I ate the nuts,' she prays. Brian was just a babe in arms at the time, and remained oblivious throughout; but Fiona, who was only three years old, became wonderfully protective of her older sibling. She wouldn't let her eat *anything* — and I mean anything — before asking us if there were nuts in it! Thankfully, Aisling is a very sensible young lady, and *never* eats a new food without first asking us whether it is safe to do so. She also carries an adrenaline syringe at all times: in her schoolbag, in the car and in the home. She is brought to friends' parties with a present in one hand and a syringe in the other. The hosts at each and every event are discreetly taken to one side for a brief but very clear instruction: NO NUTS! And if a 'hidden' nut is eaten accidentally: USE THE ADRENALINE!

What is anaphylaxis?

Anaphylaxis, or anaphylactic shock, is a term used in clinical practice to describe a rapidly progressive and potentially fatal allergic reaction. The word comes from the Greek *phulaxis*, meaning protection. *Ana*phylaxis refers to those who have 'no protection' when they meet their allergen.

A little history

The phenomenon of anaphylaxis was discovered accidentally, in 1902, by two French Nobel prizewinners, Charles Richet and Paul Jules Portier. They were studying the Portuguese man-of-war (a nasty jellyfish), and specifically the toxin in its tentacles. They hoped to develop an antidote for those who were stung by it. At first, they tried to immunise dogs by giving them a course of injections containing tiny amounts of toxin. The dogs had no problem with the first injection. However, and to the great dismay of all concerned, the dogs died very rapidly after a second injection. The scientists concluded that the first injection — far from immunising the dogs — had increased their sensitivity! The dogs were now considered to be so sensitive to toxin that they were 'without protection'. They were defenceless, they had anaphylaxis.

At this time, other doctors were busy trying to protect their patients from another threat: serious and often fatal infections, such as diphtheria and tetanus. To achieve protection, doctors vaccinated their patients with specific antibodies. It worked very well. Recipients were rendered immune to the offending bacteria and were thus spared the ravages of infection. However, some patients died at the time of injection, *from the injection*! And so doctors discovered, much to their chagrin, that one could develop anaphylaxis to vaccines as well as to toxin.

As mentioned earlier, the Viennese paediatrician Clemens von Pirquet observed in 1906 that these patients had an *abnormal response* to the horse serum then commonly used in vaccines, and were in a state of 'altered reactivity' — they had allergy. Furthermore, he realised that the unfortunate dogs did not die from the effects of toxin per se, but from their *abnormal response* to it. So, allergy and anaphylaxis then referred to one and the same thing.

As time went by, it became increasingly clear that virtually any substance, from peanut to penicillin, could induce anaphylaxis/allergy in susceptible people. It also became clear that there were degrees of sensitivity, and that not all states of 'altered reactivity' were fatal, or even nearly fatal. In clinical practice, therefore, we now make a distinction between anaphylaxis and allergy. Anaphylaxis refers to fatal or potentially fatal reactions; whereas allergy, as a broader term, refers to any hypersensitive reaction, regardless of its severity.

There is, however, something of a grey area here, an uncertainty in our science and in our clinical practice. We can all understand the difference between fatal and non-fatal, but how are we to judge the 'potentially fatal'? The sad truth is that we have no clear dividing line between 'just a bad allergy' and 'a slight touch of anaphylaxis'. There is a need, therefore, to exercise careful clinical judgment when dealing with each individual patient.

Why is anaphylaxis so deadly?

As we have seen, it is not the allergen per se which causes damage, but the body's abnormal response to it is catastrophic. This is true of all allergic disorders, but never more so than in the case of anaphylaxis. There seems to be another factor at play here, an 'accelerator' of some sort, which drives the allergy to frightening extremes. We don't know what this accelerator is, but we know that it's there, and we know that it's lethal.

To understand this more fully, we will need to know something about the underlying mechanisms involved. To this end, let us start with the 'final common pathway', and work backwards. The final common pathway, in this context, refers to a series of events which take place in the body during an anaphylactic reaction — whatever the cause of the reaction. We come yet again to our old friend (or enemy, as the case may be), the mast cell. And we meet, for the first time, its cousin the basophil. Simply put, the basophil is a mast cell which floats freely in the bloodstream. Both of these cells contain numerous potent chemicals. When they burst (degranulate) they release their potent load into the surrounding tissues and bloodstream. Once emptied, they can produce new chemicals at a ferocious pace, thus ensuring a continuous reaction.

'But hold it right there!' you may say, 'Isn't that what happens in allergic asthma, rhinitis, urticaria, angioedema, and so on?' And, of course, you would be right. That's exactly what happens in all type 1 forms of allergy. The difference in anaphylaxis is the 'accelerating factor' alluded to above. Let me illustrate this. Kevin is a ten-year-old boy with a history of asthma. His symptoms are well controlled because he takes his medication regularly and he has, with a little help, figured out his allergic and non-allergic triggers. His only other problem is that he is allergic to eggs. If he eats egg two days in a row he gets hives (urticaria). If he eats egg one day, avoids it the next, and eats it again on the third day, he gets no hives. The skin and blood tests confirm that he is sensitive to eggs, but he has never had a major reaction to them.

Okay, so Kevin has an allergy. Now compare that with another ten-year-old boy, Damien. He has no history of asthma, nor of any other allergic disease for that matter. He came to the Allergy Clinic because he broke out in hives and vomited violently after eating an egg. His mother assumed he was allergic to eggs and kept him away from them. Damien needed no

114

encouragement to comply with this restriction, for he noticed a tingling rash on his face whenever eggs were being fried in the vicinity! However, some time later he again broke out in hives, vomited, and this time started to wheeze. He was puzzled because he hadn't eaten, or even been near, eggs — but he had just eaten fish fingers, and, although he didn't know it, fish fingers contain egg.

Damien has anaphylaxis. He has something other than what we might call 'a simple allergy'. He has an accelerating mechanism at work in his system which drives a fulminant reaction *throughout his entire system* (that's why we call them *systemic reactions*). This happens whenever he comes across even *minute* amounts of allergen. Think about it. He comes across the *smell* of eggs in the frying pan and he gets symptoms. We are talking *molecules* of allergen here, not milligrams or ounces. Yet these few molecules can start a devastating cascade of allergic events throughout his system. You think I'm exaggerating? At the time of writing, an unfortunate visitor to a London restaurant collapsed with fatal anaphylaxis as a waiter walked past with a sizzling fish dish. He was known to be allergic to fish. That's what I mean by an accelerator, and that's what makes anaphylaxis so deadly.

Come back for a moment to the mast cell and basophil. The release of their potent load gives rise to the symptoms of allergy. As we have seen, if they degranulate in the nose we get rhinitis, in the chest we get asthma, in the skin we get urticaria, and so forth. However, if an accelerator is present, the cells degranulate throughout the entire system, and not just where allergen has reached. This is how it happens:

1. Something triggers the mast cells and basophils.
2. They degranulate, pouring their potent chemicals into the tissues and bloodstream.
3. These chemicals have a direct effect on blood vessels, making them dilate.
4. Dilated blood vessels are 'leaky', and allow fluid to escape from the bloodstream into the soft tissues and other organs, including the liver, intestine, lungs and brain.
5. These chemicals also exert a direct effect on smooth muscle, making it contract.
6. Smooth muscles in the bronchial tubes, intestine and womb go into spasm.

The symptoms and signs of anaphylaxis arise directly from the above:

- hives and swellings in the skin (urticaria and angioedema)
and/or
- sneezing (and other symptoms of rhinitis)
and/or
- watery eyes (and other symptoms of conjunctivitis)
and/or
- wheezing (and other symptoms of acute asthma)
and/or
- difficulty taking a breath
and/or
- hoarseness of voice
and/or
- abdominal pain
and/or
- vomiting and diarrhoea (which may be bloody)
and/or
- anxiety, fainting and convulsions
and/or
- irregular heartbeats, heart attack and, ultimately, cardiac arrest

Anaphylaxis is so deadly because of its effects on the airways, the heart and the brain. Let's take a closer look at these.

The airway in anaphylaxis

The airway may be threatened at several levels: (i) the throat and voice box, (ii) the bronchial tubes and (iii) the lungs themselves.

(i)   As we have seen in a previous chapter, space is limited in the throat and voice box. When the swellings of angioedema occur in these places they can easily obstruct the airway. Indeed, sometimes the airway is completely obstructed. The symptoms of obstruction include a sensation of swelling in the throat, difficulty taking a breath, difficulty swallowing, drooling from the mouth, hoarseness of speech, noisy breathing and, when obstruction is complete, absolute inability to breathe.

(ii)   Anaphylaxis affects the bronchial tubes in an asthmatic sort of way. They swell, go into spasm and produce thick mucus — all of which narrows the airway. The symptoms include cough, wheeze and shortness of breath. The progression of the asthmatic attack in anaphylaxis may be extremely rapid.

(iii) Finally, the lungs themselves are affected, as indeed are all internal organs. The leaky blood vessels allow fluid to pour out of the bloodstream and into the alveoli (the air sacs we talked about in chapter 5). Thus, the lungs drown in their own fluids.

The heart in anaphylaxis

The heart may also be affected in several ways:

(i) Mast cells in the heart muscle burst, causing swelling and disruption of the heart's normal rhythm.

(ii) The blood flow to the heart may be jeopardised, resulting in a heart attack.

(iii) The heart comes under further strain as the blood pressure falls. It may now beat erratically, sometimes stopping altogether — cardiac arrest!

The brain in anaphylaxis

One of the first 'brain' symptoms of anaphylaxis is a feeling of impending doom. The patient becomes anxious — even before the other symptoms of 'allergy' are manifest. Falling blood pressure may then cause a feeling of faintness, and more profound drops in pressure lead to loss of consciousness. Swelling in the brain may cause convulsions and coma.

THE END RESULT OF UNHALTED ANAPHYLAXIS IS A COMPLETE (METABOLIC) COLLAPSE OF THE SYSTEM AND DEATH.

Different types of anaphylaxis

There are several different types of anaphylaxis, all of them sharing the final common pathway just described above. Thus, they all share the same symptom complex and they carry the same risk. The final pathway is like the proverbial row of dominoes, all neatly lined up in close proximity. Knock the first one over and the whole row will fall, one by one. This is the sort of chain reaction which occurs in anaphylaxis. It does not matter how you knock the first domino, it matters only that it falls. Thus, you could blow it over, you could flick it with a finger or you could hit it with a hammer: the end result will always be the same.

As we have seen, the first domino to fall in anaphylaxis is 'mast cell and basophil degranulation'. We must now turn our attention to the triggers, the several and diverse mechanisms by which these cells burst in the first place. The triggers are as different from each other as chalk and cheese, but the symptoms will be the same, no matter what the cause. We therefore cannot distinguish one type of anaphylaxis from the next by just looking at the symptoms. It is the triggering mechanism alone which differs.

Anaphylaxis — the allergic triggers

The most common type of anaphylaxis involves IgE, the allergy antibody. In this scenario, when a patient becomes sensitised to an allergen, they produce a very specific clone of IgE. This IgE will react exclusively to that allergen — the only exception to the rule being the phenomenon of cross-reactivity (see p. 55). The IgE antibodies are stationed (mostly) on mast cell membranes (walls) throughout the body. When the allergen comes floating by, the IgE reaches out an arm and grabs it. If any two IgEs grab the allergen in this way, they are said to be 'bridged' (joined together by allergen). Bridged IgEs rapidly change shape and, in so doing, trigger the mast cell to degranulate! It's a bit like one of those strongrooms found in banks: two keys must be turned simultaneously to unlock the door.

Anaphylaxis — the non-allergic triggers

Several other triggers of anaphylaxis have been identified. In each of these cases, mast cells and basophils are triggered by mechanisms *other than IgE*. However, these mechanisms, by virtue of their complexity, are beyond the scope of this book. Nevertheless, you may be interested in this one.

Exercise-induced anaphylaxis

The body releases some very potent chemicals during physical exercise. These can trigger mast cell degranulation in susceptible individuals. Sometimes degranulation will occur only in the presence of a 'dormant allergy'; at other times it will occur without any other apparent reason. Ken, for instance, is a track and field athlete, well used to training, and motivated by aspirations to stardom. He thought his dreams were over when he discovered that he was no longer able to train without getting violently ill. The first thirty minutes were no problem, but symptoms came on shortly after that, depending to some extent on his training schedule. He would first notice a tingling sensation on his lips, then he would feel nauseated and vomit. Within minutes of vomiting he would have to dash to the toilet with diarrhoea. But the exertion of the dash only added to his woes, so sometimes he made it and sometimes he didn't. If he rested, his symptoms would gradually subside.

His only clue that allergy may have been responsible was the tingling on his lips, so he came to the Allergy Clinic. I asked Ken to fast for five hours, and then to train again (under supervision). This time he was able to run for forty-five minutes, non-stop and at quite a pace, stopping only because he was tired and not because he was ill. Needless to say, he was delighted with himself. We had now demonstrated that his anaphylaxis (for that's what it was) was related in some way to food. He ate a very healthy diet, including daily doses of his favourite snack: apple and celery salad. And celery, for some unknown reason, is frequently implicated in this sort of food-related exercise-induced anaphylaxis. Ken can now train as hard as he likes *as long as he avoids celery.*

The converse phenomenon is also true, as demonstrated recently by a case report from a colleague. He described a woman in her fifties who was very fond of dancing. She developed exercise-induced anaphylaxis on the dance floor, but only after drinking brandy! She could dance all night if she didn't drink and she could drink all night if she didn't dance. (Don't try this one at home!)

Declan wasn't so lucky. He had played squash for several years without incident. Recently, however, he started to itch after some twenty minutes of play. He put it down to a 'sweat rash' and tried to ignore it. But, as the season progressed, he ran into more trouble: he noticed that the itch appeared after five minutes of play, and that it was getting worse. The day came when the itch 'went mad altogether', and this time he broke out in swellings all over his body. Not only that, but his tongue and lips were swollen, he had difficult wheezy breathing, he couldn't drink and he was hoarse. In other words, he had anaphylaxis. We got him to exercise after a five-hour fast, but he got symptoms within minutes and had to stop. His exercise-induced anaphylaxis is not related to food. He has either (i) started to release too many potent chemicals in his body during exercise, or (ii) developed an intolerance to the normal levels that we all produce. The bottom line is that Declan must now avoid physical exertion, full stop.

Who gets it?

Anybody can get anaphylaxis. A history of allergy in the family or a history of allergy in the patient are *not* definite risk factors. Similarly, there is no evidence that sex, age, race or occupation are associated with the condition. However, patients with a history of asthma are likely to have more severe anaphylaxis when they do get it.

Will they grow out of it?

No. Although many young children grow out of their allergies, those who have had a life-threatening reaction should be considered anaphylactic for life.

What causes it?

Anaphylaxis can be induced by many diverse triggers, including, but not exclusively, the following.

Injected triggers

- Penicillin
- Insulin, vaccines or any other injected medicine
- X-ray dyes
  These are used in radiology to obtain useful pictures of blood vessels and other structures. Blockage in the coronary arteries, for instance, can be visualised in this way. Some 5 to 8 per cent of patients react adversely to the dye, but the vast majority of these are minor reactions and of no clinical significance. However, one in every thousand patients can expect a more serious anaphylactic reaction.*
- Blood transfusions
  Although this is very rare, some patients will develop anaphylactic reactions to blood, even when it's properly cross-matched to their own blood group.‡
- Anaesthetic agents
  These may have a direct effect on mast cell degranulation in susceptible patients. An anaesthetist can expect at least 1 anaphylactic reaction to occur in every 50,000 general anaesthetics administered (although the true figure could be as high as 1 in 3,500).
- Skin-prick testing
- Insect stings or bites

---

*The mechanism here, for those who wish to know, is the 'complement pathway'.
‡The mechanism here is the 'alternative complement pathway'.

Ingested triggers

- Medicines
  Some drugs, such as aspirin and morphine, exert a direct effect on mast cells; others may induce allergic reactions involving IgE.
- Foods: seafood, nuts, berries and legumes; but virtually any food can do it!
- Food additives
- Drinks

Inhaled triggers

- Food dusts
- Penicillin dusts
- Other occupational dusts
- Latex (absorbed into powder on surgical gloves)

Contact triggers

- Latex
- Seminal fluid
- Topical medication, e.g. fluorescein dye
- Others: mercurochrome, lidocaine, chlorhexidine, formaldehyde, milk (casein), castor bean

Other triggers

- Exercise
- Cold exposure
  This can degranulate mast cells in susceptible individuals, especially after immersion in cold water (see p. 47).

Anaphylaxis — cause unknown

Finally, there is a small group of patients who suffer from recurrent bouts of anaphylaxis in whom no trigger can be found. We refer to this as 'idiopathic' anaphylaxis, meaning 'of unknown origin'. This diagnosis (or lack of diagnosis) is entertained only after a thorough investigation has failed to identify a trigger.

Are there any complications?

In spite of the foregoing, it must be said that recovery from anaphylaxis is usually rapid and complete, taking no more than twelve hours in most cases. Occasionally, the anaphylaxis may be prolonged and require continuous treatment (the record is twenty-three days in intensive care!). Nevertheless, although most patients recover from their anaphylaxis, deaths can and do occur.

What can we do about it?

There are a few imperatives that I would like to bring to the attention of patients who have experienced a life-threatening reaction:

1. Every effort should be made to identify your anaphylactic trigger.
2. You should avoid your anaphylactic trigger at all times in the future.
3. Register with Medic Alert® (see appendix 2).
4. You must receive the correct treatment without delay if you are ever accidentally exposed to your anaphylactic trigger again.

1. Identify the trigger

Identifying the trigger is not always as easy as it sounds. Notwithstanding, a detailed clinical history with a specialist doctor, together with blood tests and, if necessary, skin tests, will reveal the majority of triggers. Patients often know if a food is responsible because the reactions are usually so rapid and dramatic. Nevertheless, they should assume nothing until we have obtained objective evidence of allergy. So, having decided on a suspect, or perhaps a shortlist of suspects, we should proceed to the blood test. This is a very straightforward test in which we measure the levels of IgE in blood, and determine what it is reacting to. Admittedly, the test is not without fault, but it is very useful nonetheless. This is an extremely important point. Sometimes the test will come back 'negative' for an allergen when the patient is in fact highly allergic to that allergen. We call these 'false negatives'. *A negative blood test, therefore, should never be relied upon to exclude an allergy!*

False positive blood tests are much less common, but they do also occur. In particular, the allergist must guard against the temptation to blame an allergen simply because it shows up in the blood. It must be demonstrated that this allergen is relevant to the anaphylaxis, and not just an incidental finding. In other words, even positive blood tests may need to be confirmed by other means, especially if there is reasonable doubt as to their relevance. So, if the blood test is negative, or 'borderline', or if the positive test is of doubtful significance, we should proceed to skin tests. These should always be done with the utmost care, for you may have noticed above that skin-prick tests are a known trigger for anaphylaxis in their own right. Therefore, **do not be tempted to do this at home!** (See chapter 17 for more details on skin tests.)

If the skin tests are also negative, we then move on cautiously to more direct challenges. This involves smearing the suspect food onto a lip and waiting to see the response. If there is no reaction, a minute amount is given by mouth and we wait again for ten or fifteen minutes. If there is no reaction we give a little more by mouth, and wait. We continue in this manner until the patient either has a reaction or is able to eat normal quantities of the suspect food without adversity — in which case that food is no longer a suspect.

Some recent cases come to mind by which we can illustrate some of these points. The first is a policeman who developed a fulminant itchy rash over his whole body ten minutes after licking peanut butter from a spoon. He also developed a pounding headache and felt ill. Naturally, he suspected that peanut had caused his trouble. The blood test came back negative, so we proceeded to skin tests. At first, we diluted peanut to a 1 in 15,000 solution, placed it on his forearm, and pricked the underlying skin through the droplet. Nothing happened. Then we repeated the test with a 1 in 3,000 dilution, and again nothing happened. We moved thus, in stepwise fashion, to higher concentrations until we reached the pure 1 in 1 extract; then we injected his skin; and finally we gave him a peanut to eat. Nothing happened. He ate the whole packet of peanuts and still did not react. Whatever it was that caused his rash, it wasn't peanut!

This case is in stark contrast to our next patient, Seán, an eighteen-year-old with a long-standing history of suspected egg allergy. I say 'suspected' because he had never been fully assessed. He was admitted to hospital when he was a baby, with asthma, diarrhoea, vomiting and a rash. His mother suspected that he had an allergy because his symptoms started after a meal which consisted, amongst other things, of egg. Seán, for his part, reckoned that eggs had 'always been a problem' for him. His eyes would stream, his skin would itch and he would start to wheeze if eggs were broken in the kitchen. At least, he thought it was the eggs, but he wasn't really sure. In any case, eggs had been banned from the house ever since. The question now being asked was 'Does Seán really have an egg allergy, and if he does, will he have to avoid egg in his adult life?' Seán's blood test was negative, so we proceeded cautiously to skin tests. A drop of egg white and another of egg yolk were placed on his forearm and pricked. Nothing happened. Then we gave him a tiny injection of egg into the skin. Within five minutes he had produced a swelling the size of a golf ball. Seán's blood test was a false negative. He is allergic to eggs, and he should be considered anaphylactic for the rest of his life. Meanwhile, I asked Seán to stay in the Allergy Clinic for two hours, as a precaution. The swelling subsided during this time and no other symptoms developed. It was now safe for him to go home.

And then there was Imelda, a woman in her forties with asthma. She was doing quite well until she got an asthmatic attack at a restaurant. She suspected a food because she had been so well before the meal, and became so ill during it. The list of potential candidates was long, so we started to screen. It wasn't long before we came to kiwi. Imelda started to wheeze, and developed hives on her arm within five minutes of the skin test. She was given a preloaded adrenaline syringe for future emergencies, instructed in its use, and advised never to eat kiwi again. There is a sequel to this story, which you will read about presently.

Finally, idiopathic anaphylaxis presents the greatest challenge of all. By definition, we are unable to find a trigger in this condition. It is possible that it represents a disease in its own right, and that some patients just have spontaneous anaphylaxis. But it is equally possible that we simply haven't put our finger on the trigger. Take the case of a fish handler who was getting repeated attacks of unexplained anaphylaxis. He was not allergic to fish, but frequently collapsed at work. Then some clever doctor looked more closely at the fish, and found that his patient was highly sensitive to Anisakis simplex — a fish parasite! Or the case of the man who carved items out of deer antler, who also frequently collapsed at work but was found to be 'not allergic' to deer horn dust. However, it was eventually realised that he was allergic to deer horn but only after it was treated with specific chemicals. Other patients have reacted to hidden allergens in a similar way. So, if you have 'idiopathic' anaphylaxis never stop searching for the trigger!

2. Avoid the anaphylactic trigger

You simply cannot afford to relax on this one, particularly in view of the fact that *subsequent reactions tend to be more severe.* Therefore, the old adage that prevention is better than cure certainly applies here. You will need expert guidance on hidden sources of allergen from a doctor with an interest, and/or from a dietician with an interest. For example, it is always hazardous for the anaphylactic patient to eat outside of their own home. They can never be sure that the caterer understands the need for extreme care, and this is where we come back to Imelda. She went to a restaurant only two weeks after receiving her adrenaline syringe. She told the waitress about her problem with kiwi, and then ordered her meal. She politely asked that the chef use a clean knife when preparing her melon. She also requested that the melon be prepared on a clean cutting board. The melon arrived with two thin slices of apple to one side. Everything looked fine and Imelda put some apple into her mouth. She collapsed within seconds, unconscious, and unable to help herself to the adrenaline. Her husband, who had familiarised himself with the adrenaline, took it out of her handbag and injected her straight away. She came round immediately, spat out the food, and inspected its contents. There was a very tiny piece of kiwi on the underside of the sliced apple.

Other patients have stumbled upon their allergen in unrecognised forms: peanut in satay sauce, buckwheat in wheat burger, shrimp in a Chinese sauce, walnut in a lamb stew, peanut in cheesecake, egg in fishfingers, etc. Tragically, some of these patients died as a result. They died for two reasons. In the first place, **they were caught unawares** when they were eating out. Secondly, **they did not have their adrenaline syringe** with them at the time. *Do not put your life into the hands of a caterer, and never leave home without adrenaline.*

3. Register with Medic Alert

Medic Alert is an emergency identification system for people with hidden medical conditions, including anaphylaxis. When you register with Medic Alert, your medical details will be recorded (confidentially) in a central database. You will also be offered a neck pendant or bracelet which bears an internationally recognised medical emblem, together with a phone number to the central database, and brief details of your medical condition, e.g. 'Anaphylaxis to penicillin'. Thus, medical staff are immediately made aware of your condition. The Medic Alert foundation is an international non-profit-making registered charity.

4. Emergency treatment for anaphylaxis

It is impossible to predict the severity or outcome of a given reaction at the onset of symptoms: some will turn out to be relatively mild, and others will result in coma or death within seconds of trigger exposure. Remember, subsequent reactions tend to get worse. In general, mortality correlates with

- the speed of symptom onset
- the severity and duration of symptoms, and
- whether adrenaline was given early in the course of treatment

We can do nothing about the speed or severity of symptoms when they strike, but we can do something about adrenaline. It is imperative that correct therapy be administered as soon as possible, regardless of the trigger or of the severity of symptoms. There is no time for delay, and **there is no substitute for adrenaline in the treatment of anaphylaxis.**

Adrenaline

Adrenaline is the only therapeutic agent with immediate anti-anaphylactic effects. It inhibits the degranulation of mast cells and basophils. It also (i) increases blood flow, (ii) increases blood pressure, (iii) relieves spasm in the bronchial tubes, and (iv) reduces swelling in the internal organs. In other words, it reverses all of the final common pathway events. Antihistamines and steroids, on the other hand, have no such immediate effect and THEY SHOULD NOT BE RELIED UPON TO TREAT ANAPHYLAXIS. However, they *may* help to prevent late-phase reactions (see below), and this is the only reason for using them in the treatment of anaphylaxis.

Anyone who has had a life-threatening anaphylaxis, or a life-threatening angioedema in the airway, should be given a pre-loaded adrenaline syringe for use in an emergency. In fact, they should have at least two syringes immediately available to them, and another two in the local pharmacy for immediate replacement (if the need arises). Those who live or work in remote areas should have four syringes. This is the only way to ensure that adrenaline is given as early as possible in the course of treatment. Possible exceptions to this rule of thumb are patients with thyroid disease, heart disease or high blood pressure.

Several preloaded syringes for the emergency treatment of anaphylaxis are available on prescription. The adult ones contain 0.3 mg of adrenaline, the paediatric ones 0.15 mg. They are deliberately modest doses, and because they're modest they're safe. Thus, otherwise healthy patients should always remember that there is *far greater benefit than risk* in giving themselves adrenaline during anaphylaxis. If the first dose wears off after a while, give yourself another one. Indeed, the dose can be repeated at ten-minute intervals if need be.

Anaphylaxis, as you well know, is dramatic and frightening. Therefore, be sure that you are familiar with your preloaded syringe. You don't want to be fumbling about with it when you're in a hurry. Practise regularly with a special training (dummy) device. Also, make sure that your nearest and dearest are familiar with the device — they may need to help you in an emergency.

After adrenaline, what?

Adrenaline is not a substitute for medical care, it buys you time to get medical care. As soon as you have given yourself the injection you *go to hospital*. If the first dose of adrenaline wears off on the way, take a second. When you reach hospital, go straight to the Accident and Emergency Department, tell them you have anaphylaxis, and show them your Medic Alert card (or bracelet/necklace). Do not sit politely in the waiting room — this is an emergency, and you need immediate care. You should be admitted to hospital for a period of observation, even after apparently full recovery. This is because the anaphylaxis could flare up again within the next eight hours — in spite of the fact that you have no further contact with your trigger. Indeed, some 25 per cent of patients with anaphylaxis may experience this 'late-phase' event.

And then what?

Once you have recovered from your anaphylaxis you should review the event with your doctor or allergist, renew your adrenaline prescription immediately, and ask yourself some questions. How did this happen? Did I relax my guard? Did I come across my allergen/trigger in some unexpected way? What can I learn from this that will help me prevent future accidental exposures?

But I'm scared stiff!

Anaphylaxis can cause great anxiety. This is perfectly under-standable, of course, and even justified. Survivors have, after all, experienced a brush with death. Knowing what caused the ana-phylaxis will help to allay fear, for you can take precautions to avoid it in the future. But spare a thought for those with idio-pathic anaphylaxis — they do not know what to do, or what to avoid. They have to wait for another episode to get another clue. If idiopathic attacks are frequent the patient should be offered continuous oral steroids to help ward off the attacks.

I advise my patients to face their fear in the following man-ner, and this applies to all forms of anaphylaxis. Firstly, acknowledge that your fear is perfectly rational. You have good cause to be afraid. Now construct a small cabinet in your mind. Place the trigger, together with your fear of the trigger, into the cabinet. Alongside it, place your supply of preloaded adrenaline. Now you can close the door, and keep the fear com-partmentalised. As long as you have your adrenaline, you have every chance of survival. Even patients with idiopathic ana-phylaxis can derive some comfort from this.

Could it be anything else?

Acute anaphylaxis is usually a straightforward diagnosis. However, the clinical presentations of anaphylaxis are varied. In the extreme, anaphylaxis may present as a sudden loss of con-sciousness without the telltale signs of allergy. This is a chal-lenge for doctors, for they must now consider the possibility of anaphylaxis in any unconscious patient. Other confusing pre-sentations may include vomiting and bloody diarrhoea. Who would expect these to be allergic in origin when they are so often caused by other disorders? Similarly, sudden airway obstruction may be mistaken for choking, and anaphylactic asthma may be treated as 'ordinary' asthma. So, as you can see, it is more likely that anaphylaxis will be underdiagnosed than overdiagnosed.

A word about panic attacks and pseudo-anaphylaxis

Panic attacks are episodes of severe anxiety, in which patients experience a whole range of physical and mental symptoms. The attack starts with a feeling of impending doom, and pro-gresses to a thumping heartbeat, shortness of breath, chest pain, light-headedness, pins and needles, and a feeling of faintness.

Nobody dies from a panic attack.

Admittedly, some panic symptoms also occur in anaphylaxis. However, the attending doctor can distinguish the severe systemic collapse of anaphylaxis from the *feeling* of systemic collapse that accompanies panic. Some patients, unfortunately, become obsessed with the notion that they have anaphylaxis, not panic, and no amount of reassurance from the allergist can convince them otherwise. That's a pity, because these patients are obviously suffering and they are not getting (or accepting) the most appropriate treatment. Rather, they spend their time going from one panic attack to another, all the time searching for an anaphylactic trigger that does not exist.

SECTION 4

Food Intolerance

10 Allergy or Intolerance: What's the Difference?

CASE HISTORY

Carmel was a 48-year-old teacher. She had a miserable life, dogged as it was by constant illness. The day she came to see me was a relatively good day, she explained, but she was plagued with symptoms even as she spoke. She was tired all the time, she had no energy, and she had one sore throat after another. 'I've even got one now,' she protested, in obvious discomfort. She took a moment to massage her throat, and continued with her story. 'My bowels are giving me gyp, and I have pains all over my body, and — ' she hesitated, as if she had suddenly realised something. She just sat there for a while gazing at the floor. Then, rather nervously, she raised an inquisitive eyebrow in my direction. No, I did not think she was mad, I reassured her; and I asked her to tell me more. It quickly became clear that Carmel had a multitude of symptoms, apparently unrelated. She had pains in her muscles and joints; her fingers and ankles were often swollen; she had mouth ulcers, bloating of the abdomen, constipation, abdominal pain and an itchy bottom; her sleep pattern was all over the place, her concentration was poor and her libido was low. Furthermore, her skin had 'gone to pot', especially just before a period. She had other premenstrual symptoms: her breasts were sore and she was particularly cranky for a week or so leading up to a period. As is so often the case, Carmel's previous investigations had drawn a blank, and she had been told that she was 'just depressed'. But Carmel would have none of it. 'Look,' she said, 'every time I eat wheat my throat flares up, and when I eat sugar I get depressed. What I want to know is could it be an allergy?'

133

Could it be an allergy?

Now there's a question that needs to be answered, for if Carmel does have an allergy, or several allergies, she could expect to find relief from her symptoms by avoiding the thing(s) she is allergic to. A blood test for allergy was performed and came back negative. However, it would be quite wrong to dismiss the possibility of allergy on this basis. Blood tests for allergy *detect only IgE allergies*; they do not reveal other kinds of allergy. This being the case, Carmel was put on the Low Allergy Diet. She was advised to eat ten prescribed foods for a period of ten days. By the tenth day she felt better than she had done for years. All of her symptoms had disappeared. When she expanded her diet again she reacted adversely to many of her staple foods. To cut a long story short, Carmel had multiple food intolerance.

Polysymptomatics

Carmel is not unusual, there are many like her who suffer for years on end with puzzling and debilitating symptoms. They have been on the merry-go-round of negative investigations, they have tried various medical treatments, and ultimately they are at risk of being dismissed. Some of them are labelled neurotic or anxious; others are told they are depressed; and a few are said to be hypochondriacs. They can see the poorly disguised heartsinking look on their doctor's face when they present with yet another baffling symptom, and yet another entry for the case notes which, at this stage, are as thick as a telephone directory. Many of them will give up going to their doctor altogether for fear they will be considered 'mad'. The true nature of their illness lies buried in a jungle of *apparently* unrelated symptoms, and it lies there, hidden, for years, until someone finally decides to look for it! It must be said that some of us are neurotic and anxious, and many of us do suffer from depression and/or hypochondriasis. We must also recognise that these disturbed mental states do give rise to physical symptoms. It is important therefore to keep an open mind in all of this. But my plea is that psychiatric diagnoses should be made only in the presence of a positive history of psychiatric illness; and they should never be used to fob off symptoms that are otherwise difficult to solve. The most common mistake in medicine is to assume that an illness is psychological when it isn't. The symptoms of food intolerance are a classical example of this.

Allergy or intolerance: what's the difference?

So, Carmel did not have allergy, but she did have food intolerance, and that begs a question: what's the difference between allergy and intolerance? Let me first summarise what we have already covered. We have defined allergy as a hypersensitive reaction to something otherwise harmless in the environment. Then, in chapter 2, we described four different types of hypersensitivity reaction. These all involve, *and can be seen to involve*, components of the immune system, namely IgE, other immunoglobulins, and immune cells. In all of these cases, we can understand much of the underlying mechanisms, and we can measure them in the laboratory. They are, without doubt, immune reactions. The purist would maintain that allergy, as a descriptive term, should be reserved for these mechanisms alone; and that all other (non-immune) adverse reactions should be called by another name, such as 'sensitivity' or 'intolerance'. Other doctors, equally clever, argue that von Pirquet's original concept of allergy was much broader than this, encompassing any state of 'altered reactivity', regardless of the mechanism. It does not matter to them if the mechanism defies understanding or measurement; it matters only that the patient reacts to something otherwise harmless in the environment.

Now, I know it all sounds a bit academic, but it does explain why there's so much confusion about. Personally, I have a great deal of sympathy with the former view, but I am also swayed by the everyday language of my patients. If they think they react to something, they tell me they're 'allergic to it', and they care not a whit whether I can understand it, measure it or explain it! Nevertheless, we must acknowledge the obvious difference that exists between these two kinds of 'allergy'. One involves the immune system and causes inflammation; the other does not. In clinical practice, then, we refer to all non-immune food reactions as food intolerance. Thus we have food allergy and intolerance to consider. In sections 2 and 3 we saw many examples of food allergy; in this section we will deal with food intolerance. Before we move on to specific syndromes, let us take a very brief look at some of the mechanisms by which food-intolerant reactions may occur.

1. Pharmacological activity of food

Some food reactions are the result of powerful natural substances present in food. These chemicals exert drug-like effects in our bodies. We refer to this phenomenon as 'false food allergy': false, only because it looks like an allergy, and isn't. Here are a few examples.

- Caffeine, an alkaloid drug. The most widely used foods with pharmacological activity are tea and coffee. They contain up to 80 and 150 mg of caffeine per cup respectively. An excessive consumption of caffeine may give rise to many diverse symptoms:

Anxiety	Irritability	Headaches	Weight loss
Tremor	Insomnia	Restless legs	Abdominal pain
Lethargy	Drowsiness	Rhinitis	Nausea
Depression	Sweats	Palpitations	Vomiting

- Histamine-containing foods. High levels of histamine occur naturally in some foods. This is a chemical we have already discussed at length in relation to allergic reactions. Histamine-containing foods include fermented cheeses and other foods, sausages, tinned foods (especially tinned smoked herring's eggs), sauerkraut and spinach. These foods, when eaten in excess and/or in combination, can cause:

Flare-up of eczema	Headache
Hot flushes	Urticaria
Angioedema	Abdominal pain
Thirst	Shock (rarely)

- Histamine-liberating foods. Some foods do not contain histamine, but they release histamine from mast cells in the body. This is a direct effect that does not involve IgE. Histamine-liberating foods include egg white, fish (especially shellfish), tomato, chocolate, pork, pineapple, strawberry, papaya and alcohol. They too can cause histamine symptoms.

- Vasoactive amines. Vasoactive amines are also natural components of food. They have a drug-like effect on blood vessels (vaso), making them dilate. This gives rise to blood vessel headache (migraine). Hist*amine* is one such amine. Others include phenylethyl*amine* from chocolate (fifty grams is enough to cause trouble); and tyr*amine* in cheese, yeast extract, pickled herring, banana, broad beans, liver, sausage and alcohol.

2. Enzyme deficiencies

Food is digested by special enzymes in the gut, and further broken down by enzymes in the blood. Enzyme deficiencies will give rise to symptoms by allowing a build-up of particular food components in the gut or in the blood. One example that we should all be familiar with is our relative intolerance to onions. We don't have the enzyme necessary to digest the sugar in this food. High levels of sugar then reach the large intestine, where they are fermented by resident microbes. Onions also contain a smelly disulphide. Excessive consumption of onions will therefore lead to smelly flatulence! Enzyme deficiencies may be more idiosyncratic, however. Lactose, for example, is the sugar found in milk. Some infants are born with a lactase deficiency, the enzyme by which we digest lactose. Lactose therefore builds up in the gut, causing a watery diarrhoea, and even collapse in some infants. Adults may acquire a transient lactase deficiency, especially after a bout of gastroenteritis, after intestinal surgery or as a complication of other bowel disease. Milk consumption in such circumstances will also cause diarrhoea and related symptoms. Many other enzyme deficiencies have been identified, some of them causing serious health effects until they are diagnosed and treated by a lifetime of dietary avoidance. PKU (phenylketonuria) is probably the best known of these: every infant is checked for this at birth with the heel-prick test.

3. Hormonal activity of foods

Food intolerance may also arise from foods that contain opium-like proteins. These include wheat, dairy produce and corn. This may be linked to enzyme deficiency, for the proteins should be broken down by enzyme activity in the gut, and later in the blood. Symptoms known to be associated with opium-like proteins include mood and behaviour disorders, Irritable Bowel Syndrome and water retention.

4. Toxins in food

It is hardly necessary to mention that some foods contain toxic chemicals that must be adequately degraded during cooking if they are not to cause trouble. Kidney (and other) beans, for example, should be soaked overnight and boiled for ninety minutes to break down the toxin therein. Abdominal cramps are the penalty for failing to take this precaution.

5. Sugars in food

Toddlers' diarrhoea has been linked to the consumption of apple and other fruit juices. The mechanism here is, once again, fermentation of undigested and unabsorbed sugars in the large intestine. Other symptoms include abdominal discomfort, flatulence and borborygmi (those gurgles you hear coming from your bowels). Sugar malabsorption may also affect adults.

6. More about sugars

Some people are intolerant to refined carbohydrates (sugars). Their sugar level soars immediately after eating sugar, but it then falls like a brick as the body strives to cope with the extra load. The symptoms include sweating, fatigue, weakness, hunger, disorientation, light-headedness and confusion.

7. Other components of food

Vegetables, like fruit, contain indigestible sugars, such as raffinose, and may cause a similar fermentation reaction. They also contain other active components. Flavone compounds, for example, are known to affect intestinal motility. This leads to abdominal distension and discomfort in susceptible people. Cabbage is notorious in this regard. Another fairly common problem is fatty food intolerance. Fats are digested by bile from the gall bladder. They can cause a great deal of trouble for patients with gall bladder disease.

8. Unknown immune reactions

It must be said that the immune system does not sit idly by during all food-intolerant reactions. Desensitisation for food intolerance is very effective and works by re-educating the immune system in some way (see chapter 18). This suggests that food intolerance may involve the immune system after all. We know that IgE and other antibodies are not involved, but perhaps other immune mechanisms are. For example, a food may cause the release of immune chemicals not yet measured routinely in hospital laboratories. As you will discover in chapter 16, these chemicals have profound effects on the brain and hormone systems, and may thus easily give rise to symptoms. If this turns out to be true, we shall have to redefine allergy yet again! The science of food intolerance is in its infancy, and we still have so much to learn. We have made a start, however. In the following chapters you will see that food intolerance, by whatever mechanism, is responsible for a great many ills; and that lasting relief can be obtained by discovering what your particular 'allergies' are.

11   *Allergy and the Gut*

The healthy gut

The function of the gastrointestinal tract is to ingest, digest, and absorb nutrients from food. Each specialised structure along the tract has its own part to play in this vital process.

- The mouth:

  takes food into the body, chews it, mixes it with saliva, and initiates the swallow reflex. We eat 100 tons of food during a lifetime.

- Saliva:

  lubricates food, and contains digestive enzymes which start to work on the starch component of food straight away. We produce in excess of one litre of saliva every day.

- The gullet (oesophagus):

  accepts the swallow reflex and carries on one of its own to transport food down to the stomach.

- The stomach:

  stores and churns food with its own juices before releasing it, bit by bit, into the small intestine.

- The small intestine:

  accepts food from the stomach, bile from the liver, and digestive enzymes from the pancreas. This mixture then travels at a rate of 1 cm per minute, thus facilitating the absorption of water and nutrients along its entire and considerable length.

- The large intestine (colon):

  accepts food from the small intestine, absorbs some water and nutrients, and stores and lubricates the waste matter

	(faeces) until a convenient moment for disposal.
• The anus:	prevents faeces from dribbling by its muscular (sphincter) tone.
• The stool:	The whole process of digestion and absorption is so efficient that less than one-fifth of all the material entering the small intestine is eventually expelled in the stool. The smell of the stool comes from the bacterial products present therein. The normal frequency of bowel movements is quite broad, ranging from three times a day to twice a week.

In health, we are conscious only of the sensation of hunger, the pleasure of eating, the occasional passage of wind, and the call to stool. The stool itself should be well formed, brown, not excessively smelly, and of a consistency which makes it sink rather than float on the water. It should disappear with one flush of the toilet. Now compare that with the case histories which follow. Bear in mind, as you go through this chapter, that my purpose is not to give an exhaustive account of all bowel diseases, but rather to demonstrate the important role of food intolerance as a driving force behind many bowel symptoms.

1. Coeliac disease

June is a twelve-year-old girl who was brought to the Allergy Clinic by her parents. They were concerned about her listlessness, her loss of appetite, and the fact that she was having such trouble with her bowels. When asked for details, June's parents told me that her tummy was frequently bloated 'like a potbelly', and that her bowel motions were pale and very foul-smelling. When questioned further, they confirmed that the stool was greasy and bulky, that it floated on the water, and that it hardly ever disappeared with one flush of the loo. June also volunteered that she suffered from bellyache, especially when she felt the call to stool. Hospital investigations confirmed that she was suffering from **coeliac disease**. However, some symptoms persisted in spite of the fact that she kept to her gluten-free diet. We then put her through the Low Allergy Diet and found, to everyone's relief, that she became symptom-free. Subsequent challenges revealed that she was intolerant not only to gluten but to milk. Thus, some of her symptoms were due to gluten sensitivity, and others were due to non-gluten foods.

What is coeliac disease?

Coeliac disease is a disorder characterised by damage to the lining of the small intestine. The damage is caused by a hypersensitive reaction to gluten — the protein found in wheat and rye. Gluten is also closely related to avenin, a protein found in oats, and hordein, a protein found in barley. In practice, we refer to all of these proteins collectively, if rather inaccurately, as 'gluten'. The immune system reacts against components of gluten, and destroys the lining — the absorptive surface — of the small intestine. As a result, the absorptive capacity of the intestine is greatly reduced and important dietary components are not absorbed into the body. This malabsorption, as we call it, affects proteins, carbohydrates and fats, as well as some essential vitamins and minerals. This leads on directly to nutritional deficiencies and abnormal stools.

Nutritional deficiencies in coeliac disease

The essential nutrients which a coeliac may not absorb include vitamin B12, folic acid and (less commonly) iron. These deficiencies result in anaemia (a low blood count). Other nutrients at risk include the B vitamins, vitamin K and potassium. Such deficiencies result, respectively, in tongue and mouth changes, bruising and weakness. Finally, vitamin D and calcium malabsorption may result in soft, tender bones and muscle weakness.

Stool changes in coeliac disease

Think about this for a moment. If what we eat is not absorbed it passes unchanged through the small intestine into the large, eventually appearing in the stool. In coeliac disease, it is the undigested fats, in particular, which alter the nature of the stool. They impart a greasy, bulky and frothy appearance. The fatty stool is also lighter than normal, and this explains why it floats on the water, and why it is so difficult to flush away. Furthermore, this very abnormal stool alters both the nature and the activity of resident bacterial colonies, allowing bacterial overgrowth to occur. This results in excessive gas production and foul-smelling stools.

The symptoms of coeliac disease are easily understood from the foregoing, and include:

- pale smelly stools, which are bulky, greasy and frothy
- bloated abdomen
- diarrhoea or, less commonly, constipation
- smelly flatulence
- abdominal colic
- vomiting
- poor appetite
- weight loss
- lethargy and misery

Who gets it?

Coeliac disease may appear for the first time in either childhood or adulthood. The vast majority of affected children are diagnosed before they are two years old, and the remainder are picked up by their fifth birthday. The disease may also present in later life, particularly during the third to sixth decades. As one might expect, coeliac disease occurs only in those parts of the world where gluten is ingested, and particularly amongst populations of European origin. The highest documented incidence of coeliac disease is in the west of Ireland.

Will they grow out of it?

No. Once a coeliac, always a coeliac. For this reason it is important that affected patients adhere to their gluten-free diet throughout life. Do not be lulled into a false sense of security by the apparent lessening of symptoms in the late teen and early adult years. All of the coeliac symptoms will recur sooner or later if the gluten-free diet is broken.

What causes it?

As mentioned above, we know that the immune system reacts in some way to components of gluten, destroying the lining of the small intestine in the process. We also know that there is a genetic factor involved because it is more common amongst members of the same family, and amongst those of a particular genetic make-up. However, identical twins are not always affected, and not all coeliacs share the same genetic characteristics. This means that genetic factors alone cannot explain all cases.

Furthermore, it has been extremely difficult to unravel the precise nature of the immune response in coeliac disease. Is it a type 3 hypersensitivity in which antibodies bind to gluten, form immune complexes, and damage the intestine when they are deposited there? Or is it a type 2 hypersensitivity in which gluten is bound directly to intestinal cell walls, leading to their destruction? Or, finally, is it a disease sparked off in susceptible individuals by a virus which resembles a part of the gluten molecule?

Are there any complications?

Complications in coeliac disease arise mostly in untreated cases, or when patients wittingly or unwittingly are exposed to gluten. These include:

- Anaemia
- Failure to thrive (in infants)
- Growth retardation (in children)
- Soft and tender bones (in adults)
- Rickets (in children)
- Patients with coeliac disease are at greater risk of developing other diseases in the gut. This risk may be reduced by staying on a gluten-free diet. This is another reason why patients should stay on their diet for life, and should have the benefit of regular review with their specialist.
- The normal balance between the various bacteria and yeasts in the gut may be lost, giving rise to symptoms of Gut Fermentation Syndrome (see chapter 14).
- Some coeliacs develop other food intolerance, and this may be a source of confusion for them. It explains why they fail to improve as much as they had hoped (and as much as they had been promised). They are still getting symptoms from other, non-gluten foods still present in their diet. For example, up to 15 per cent of coeliacs are also sensitive to soy.

Take Barbara, for instance. She was diagnosed a coeliac some fourteen years ago, when she was in her early thirties. She went on the gluten-free diet and many of her symptoms disappeared, but she was left with 'a lot of discomfort' in her belly. In particular, she complained of a 'sour taste' in her mouth, 'a sourness' in her stomach, and she was doing a lot of belching. Her gall bladder was checked, and it was normal. So she had another biopsy of the small intestine, and it too was normal. This confirmed her own impression of excellent compliance with the gluten-free diet, but her symptoms were still a mystery. At that stage, Barbara went on the Low Allergy Diet, and lost all of her most persistent symptoms within ten days. She was intolerant not only to gluten but to some other, non-gluten foods. This restricted her diet even further, so she is now undergoing a course of desensitisation treatment to enable her to eat the non-gluten foods again. Unfortunately, desensitisation will have no effect on her gluten sensitivity.

What can we do about it?

A lot. Obviously, the priority is to secure a reliable diagnosis. This is achieved by (i) noting a complete remission of symptoms on a gluten-free diet, (ii) noting a recurrence of symptoms when gluten is eaten after a period of abstinence, (iii) biopsy confirmation of small intestinal damage whilst eating gluten and (iv) biopsy confirmation of intestinal recovery on a gluten-free diet. Once the diagnosis is established, and for the reasons outlined above, the patient is put on a gluten-free diet for life. Symptoms should improve rapidly, especially in younger patients. Older patients may need to stay on the diet for up to a year before they derive the full benefit of doing so. Having said that, if your symptoms are slow to disappear consider the Low Allergy Diet (see chapter 17) because you may have other food intolerance as well. Apart from the social nuisance of a restricted diet, coeliac patients should lead a normal and fulfilling life.

Could it be anything else?

The diagnosis of coeliac disease is not always straightforward. It depends primarily on the typical biopsy appearance of a damaged small intestine. Other conditions which can cause the same appearance include:

- parasite infections
- other food hypersensitivities, such as to milk, fish, rice, chicken, etc.
- rare deficiencies of the immune system
- rare diseases of the bowel

A word about non-coeliac gluten intolerance

It is quite possible to be intolerant to gluten and yet not have coeliac disease. In children, the symptoms include diarrhoea and vomiting after meals and, very rarely, the passage of blood or mucus in the stool. Sometimes these symptoms are accompanied by bronchitis, rhinitis and skin rash. In adults, non-coeliac gluten intolerance causes mouth ulcers, headaches, abdominal pain, vomiting and diarrhoea. A gluten-free diet brings about rapid and sustained relief from symptoms in all cases.

2. Crohn's disease

Aideen was a 33-year-old business executive. She had always enjoyed the best of health, but then her bowels started 'acting up'. She first noticed that she was passing slimy stuff, like raw egg white, from the back passage. This could happen on its own or with the stool. She then developed abdominal cramps, and the stools became looser. Within weeks she was feeling quite unwell with loss of appetite, fatigue and joint pains. Finally, blood started to appear with every bowel motion. She was admitted to hospital and a biopsy of the intestine confirmed that she had **Crohn's disease**. She was treated in hospital with medication, and given instruction on how to administer the medication to herself at home on an ongoing basis. That worked well but Aideen still had symptoms, and besides, she wasn't happy with the notion of taking medication for any length of time. In fact, when I saw her she had stopped her medication entirely and her symptoms were beginning to flare up again. She started the Low Allergy Diet and came back for review ten days later. She was able to report a reduction in all symptoms, although they hadn't cleared completely as yet. In view of her improvement, she was willing to stay on the diet for another few days, and this time her symptoms were virtually gone. Subsequently, we challenged her intestine with various foods and, in so doing, identified which foods were safe for her, and which ones were not. It was clear that Aideen had food intolerance and that this was playing a significant part in her Crohn's disease.

What is Crohn's disease?

Crohn's disease is a chronic progressive disorder characterised by patchy inflammation of the lining of the intestinal tract. Most commonly, the small intestine is affected, and particularly the distal part thereof, i.e. the part closest to the large intestine. In up to 20 per cent of patients, patches of inflammation also occur in the large bowel. Crohn's disease may also affect other parts of the body, such as the mouth. With such damage to the absorptive surface of the intestine it is not surprising that patients with Crohn's disease suffer from malabsorption. The symptoms, which usually (but not always) start suddenly, include:

- abdominal pain (which may mimic appendicitis)
- diarrhoea, which may be bloody
- loss of appetite
- bloating of the abdomen
- fever
- anaemia
- weight loss

Who gets it?

Crohn's disease usually starts in the late teens or early twenties, but may appear up to the age of forty, and rarely after that. It is equally common in males and females, and tends to run in families.

Will they grow out of it?

Crohn's disease is usually a lifelong disorder characterised by regular exacerbations. Occasionally, a young person may recover fully from a single episode of Crohn's, especially when this presents as an 'appendicitis'. These are patients who are admitted to hospital with what everyone thinks is an acute appendicitis, only to discover after surgery that it was a bout of Crohn's disease. Finally, spontaneous remissions have been known to happen from time to time, but don't hold your breath!

What causes it?

The cause of Crohn's disease is unknown. It has been linked to a bacterium called mycobacterium paratuberculosis, but the role of this bug has not yet been widely accepted within the scientific community. Nevertheless, if future research confirms that it is responsible for the disease, an antibiotic cure may become available to us. Crohn's disease is also associated with other disorders which have a known 'autoimmune' basis, and this raises the possibility of an autoimmune process in Crohn's itself. Finally, so many cases respond to dietary manipulation that the role of food intolerance cannot be excluded as being of primary importance.

Are there any complications?

Complications are kept to a minimum by prompt diagnosis and

correct treatment. They include the following:

- Growth retardation is a risk for those whose symptoms develop slowly over months or years.
- Intestinal obstruction, in more severe cases.
- Internal abscesses (not very often).
- Fistulae sometimes form. These are 'connections' between the intestine and another organ, such as the urinary bladder or the skin. Abdominal surgery promotes the formation of fistulae, and for this reason patients with Crohn's disease should avoid surgery if at all possible.
- Perforation or internal bleeding also rarely occur.

What can we do about it?

Most cases present as an acute emergency requiring hospital admission. Once the disease is brought under control with medication, we must strive to maintain the remission with medication. Exacerbations are likely to occur from time to time. Surgery should be reserved for those cases in whom it is absolutely necessary. I would advise anyone with Crohn's disease to undergo a formal investigation for food intolerance: 70 to 80 per cent of patients can expect some degree of relief from their symptoms and, for some, this relief will be dramatic. The only reliable way to determine whether *your* Crohn's disease is aggravated by food intolerance is by means of the Low Allergy Diet outlined in chapter 17.

Could it be anything else?

Crohn's disease needs to be differentiated from other inflammatory diseases of the bowel, such as ulcerative colitis.

A word about ulcerative colitis

Ulcerative colitis is characterised by ulceration of the lining of the intestine. These inflammatory ulcers are quite different from the inflammation of Crohn's disease. However, hospital investigations are required to differentiate between the two conditions. Patients with ulcerative colitis are more likely to suffer from allergic disorders such as urticaria and rhinitis. They are also frequently intolerant to milk. In spite of these 'allergic clues', ulcerative colitis rarely improves on the Low Allergy Diet, although the occasional case will do well.

3. Irritable Bowel Syndrome

Mavis was referred to the Allergy Clinic by her surgeon. She had presented to him with a host of symptoms, including abdominal pain, bloating of the abdomen, nausea, loss of appetite, heartburn and constipation. The surgeon had taken a look inside her bowel and found it to be normal in appearance. Mavis was neither amused nor consoled! 'What's causing all my trouble, then?' she enquired defiantly. The surgeon, to his great regret, gave her the usual dietary advice for patients with constipation: it made her worse! It also made her desperate, and she was willing to try the Low Allergy Diet. Within seven days all of her symptoms faded into obscurity. 'Mind you,' she explained, 'I nearly gave up in the first few days because I got this dreadful headache, and my muscles and bones were terribly sore.' She was describing the classical withdrawal symptoms that some patients suffer when they stop eating the very thing that is making them so ill. Mavis had an **Irritable Bowel Syndrome**. In her case it was driven largely by food intolerance.

What is Irritable Bowel Syndrome?

An irritable bowel is one which, quite simply, doesn't work the way it should. It looks normal to both the naked eye and the microscope. It is therefore said to be a disorder of function, rather than a disease per se. It is probably the most common disorder seen by gastroenterology specialists in the western hemisphere. The symptoms include:

- abdominal pain . . .   which is clearly related to bowel function, being either relieved by passing a stool, or associated with altered stools

  and
- altered stool frequency . . . going to the loo too often or not often enough (constipation)

  and/or
- altered stool form . . .   too hard, too soft or even watery stools

  and/or
- altered stool passage . . .   needing to rush to the loo urgently, having to strain at stool, or a feeling of not being able to rid the rectum of all its contents

and, usually,

- passing mucus from   usually mixed in with a stool, but
  the back passage . . .   may also occur all on its own
  and, usually,
- bloating of the   or a feeling of distension and
  abdomen . . .   discomfort in the tummy

Who gets it?

Up to one-fifth of the population experience some symptoms of
Irritable Bowel Syndrome. The diagnosis is usually reserved for
adults and teenagers. Younger children who eat unhealthy diets
may experience some of the symptoms, but rarely develop the
full-blown syndrome. Babies with colic and older children with
recurrent bellyache are often food-intolerant.

Will they grow out of it?

By definition, Irritable Bowel Syndrome is a chronic and recur-
ring disorder. Many patients find that their symptoms get worse
when they are under stress, and this may well account for the
waxing and waning of symptoms in this disorder.

What causes it?

We don't know the cause of Irritable Bowel Syndrome, although
several theories have been advanced. Initially, doctors thought
that the underlying problem was one of abnormal movement
along the gastrointestinal tract. This gave rise to terms such as
'spastic colon', which implied that symptoms were related to
painful muscular spasms in the colon. However, recent research
has shown that affected patients are just more sensitive to the
normal movements which occur in their bowels — not that they
have abnormal spasms. Doctors have also been interested in the
psychological aspects of irritable bowel, and some believe it is
largely a psychological problem. By this they do not mean that
symptoms are imagined, but rather that the physical symptoms
are driven by psychological stress. They are supported in their
theory by the fact that 50 per cent of these patients have an
associated (if well-hidden) anxiety or depression; and furthermore, that two-thirds of patients will admit, when questioned,
that their irritable bowel started shortly after a 'severe social
stress', such as a bereavement, a marital breakdown, etc.
Perhaps this explains why patients treated by psychotherapy do
better in the long run than those treated by medicines alone (see
chapter 16 for more on this).

Take a minute to explore this idea of mind over matter in relation to the bowels. There is a nerve that runs from the brain straight to the gut, called the vagus nerve. Mental stress flies down this 'nervous highway', and is translated very rapidly into physical sensations. Most of us will be familiar with the feeling of 'jitters' or 'butterflies' in the stomach when we are nervous. This also explains the unpleasant phenomenon of 'trench diarrhoea' experienced by frightened soldiers in battle, and the feeling of nausea which so often accompanies states of anxiety. And having said all of that, the fact that so many patients improve significantly on the Low Allergy Diet demands respect for food intolerance as an important contributing factor in up to 70 per cent of cases.

Are there any complications?

There are no serious complications. However, some patients may find their quality of life significantly affected. Their sleep may be disturbed, and they may be unable to enjoy social gatherings around food.

What can we do about it?

Every patient with Irritable Bowel Syndrome should consider a formal investigation of their diet for food intolerance, as outlined in chapter 17. The 30 per cent who do not have food intolerance have three options, not mutually exclusive:

1. Adopt a healthy diet and bowel habit:
   - Eat a high-fibre diet: plenty of wholemeal bread, wholemeal pasta and biscuits; oats; rye; muesli and other breakfast cereals, vegetables, beans and pulses, dried fruit, and nuts.
   - Drink plenty of fluids during the day. This will help to keep the stool soft.
   - Have a good-sized breakfast and go to the loo thirty to sixty minutes later — this is often the best time of day to move the bowels.
   - Allow plenty of time for a bowel motion, don't rush it.
   - Take vigorous exercise on a daily basis — this helps to keep things moving.

2. Explore the role of stress:
   - Discover how stress affects your body.
   - Develop new strategies for coping with stress.

3. Discuss the use of specific medication with your doctor:
- Antispasmodics
- Bowel stimulants
- Stool-bulking agents

Could it be anything else?

The diagnosis of Irritable Bowel Syndrome is confidently made in many cases by a careful clinical history and physical examination. Hospital investigations are sometimes required to rule out other disorders, particularly in the older patient, and in women (whose symptoms may turn out to be gynaecological in nature). Finally, the symptoms of Irritable Bowel Syndrome overlap greatly with those of gut fermentation (see chapter 14).

12.I   Allergy and the Brain: Hyperactivity

(Attention Deficit Hyperactivity Disorder)

CASE HISTORY

John was brought to the Allergy Clinic because of concerns about his progress at school. He was seven years old at the time. His teacher had complained that his concentration was poor and that he was giddy during class. His mother added that he sometimes 'goes wild, *absolutely wild*' and that he is likely to thrash out at anyone within striking distance when he gets into one of these moods. John, for his part, was more concerned about the fact that he had frequent headache, and that he was always running to the loo with diarrhoea. He also complained of feeling tired all the time — a paradoxical symptom, given that he was always on the go and never paused for a moment's rest. During his visit, he stuck his nose into every nook and cranny of the office, mauled every valuable item on the desk, spent less than 5 per cent of the time in his chair, and was pulled back several times from expensive medical equipment. Throughout this time, he shouted several unrepeatable sentences at his mother, and interrupted our conversation frequently. John, by any reasonable standards, was suffering from hyperactivity.

Hyperactive children have long tested the patience of their parents, siblings and teachers. They have also eluded the best medical attempts to categorise and tame them! Over the years, doctors have espoused, and then rejected, countless descriptive terms for the condition. This may be because the condition is in fact a conglomeration of several different conditions with overlapping features. Thus, it is important that we agree somewhat more precisely on what it is we mean by 'hyperactivity'.

What is hyperactivity?

The most recent attempt to define hyperactivity is contained in the *Diagnostic Statistical Manual* (version IV), the reference book of the American Psychiatric Association. The preferred term for hyperactivity is now Attention Deficit Hyperactivity Disorder, or ADHD for short. The essential features of ADHD are inattention, hyperactivity and impulsivity. In the assessment of an individual with suspected ADHD, we try to quantify their attention deficit and their hyperactivity.

We give their attention (concentration) span a score. To impress us, the patient must fulfil at least six of the following nine points.

The 'inattentive' patient . . .

1. is careless (pays no attention to details)
2. does not sustain attention (concentration) for long
3. does not seem to listen to instruction
4. fails to complete tasks
5. is disorganised
6. avoids demanding tasks
7. frequently loses things
8. is easily distracted
9. is forgetful

We score the hyperactivity and impulsivity together. Again, to impress us, the patient must fulfil at least six of the following nine points.

The hyperactive/impulsive patient . . .

1. fidgets and squirms in their seat constantly
2. often leaves their seat
3. runs about and/or climbs excessively
4. finds quiet activities difficult to do
5. is always on the go, always 'driven'
6. talks excessively
7. blurts out answers before questions are finished
8. has difficulty waiting for their turn
9. often intrudes on others

Every parent who reads through these lists will recognise aspects of their own child! This is so because *every child will leave its parents totally exhausted at some stage or other in its development.* In other words, every child will put its parents through phases of extreme demand. That's normal! In contrast, the truly hyperactive child never leaves its parents with any impression other than complete exhaustion and exasperation. We should also bear in mind that there is no golden standard of behaviour that can be applied to all children as the norm to which they must conform. Thus, to label a child as 'hyperactive' may reveal more about the tolerance level of the observer than the activity levels of the child! The converse is also true, as was apparent recently when I was consulted by a rather tired and worn-out mother. She brought her son with her, another seven-year-old as it happens. She wondered whether he was hyperactive, but was by no means convinced that he was. Meanwhile, the young fellow was tracing the steps of every other hyperactive child who has graced my office: going for valuables on the desk, climbing on the couch, opening closed cupboards, shouting at his mother, etc. The same retrievals from expensive equipment, and constant vigilance over dangerous waste, were necessary throughout the consultation. 'What do you think, doctor, is he a bit hyperactive?' I had no doubt that he was, but I was unable to convince his mother that this was the case. She was extremely patient; I am not!

Hyperactivity may assume one of three subtypes: predominantly inattentive, predominantly hyperactive/impulsive, or a combination of both. To qualify for the diagnosis, these symptoms should have first appeared before the age of seven years, and should have been present for some considerable time. They must also be obvious in more than one setting, for example at home and at school. The symptoms must be severe enough to interfere with the child's social or academic functioning. Finally, we must ensure that the symptoms are not due to depression or anxiety or some other such condition.

Who gets it?

Hyperactivity is, by definition, a disorder of childhood and early adolescence. It is much more common in boys than in girls, perhaps even nine times more common. There is also a genetic link, in that the concordance rate between identical twins is very high. In other words, if one identical twin has it, the other twin is virtually certain to have it as well. Researchers in Dublin have recently identified a candidate gene for the disorder.

Interestingly, affected boys tend to display more behavioural disturbance than girls, and girls tend to display greater cognitive difficulties than boys. Thus, affected girls are likely to sit quietly in class and escape attention, whereas boys are likely to cause trouble and quickly attract attention (and treatment) to themselves. It is possible therefore that girls with the disorder are not being detected as readily as boys.

Will they grow out of it?

The outlook for hyperactive children is mixed. Most will improve substantially in their late adolescence or early adulthood. A few will remain 'fully' hyperactive for much longer, and a few will remain 'partially' hyperactive. For those who do not 'grow out of it', there is a risk of psychiatric problems in later life, such as alcoholism, depression and anxiety. These adults may also find themselves subject to emotional lability, impulsivity and violent outbursts.

Are there any complications?

There are several complications to consider.

Implications for the child

In the first place the child with attention deficit will have difficulty concentrating, and is at risk of academic failure. At the very least, they will not develop their full potential. They are also unable to function socially, and are therefore at risk of becoming socially isolated. Furthermore, they are at risk of entanglement with undesirable company. They may meet other children and adolescents who are 'in trouble' for different reasons, very often reasons of misconduct based on defiance. Before long, they could find themselves embarked on a criminal career.

Implications for others

The other siblings in the family may feel aggrieved and/or neglected. This happens because of the great drain which a hyperactive child places on its parents' energies, a drain which will always be at the expense of other children in the household. Parents struggle to strike a balance between constant confrontation on the one hand and acceptable standards of discipline on the other. Teachers quickly become frustrated because they do not have the time or resources to provide the extra help which these children need.

What can we do about it?

I would like to bring you back now to John, our seven-year-old hyperactive boy with headaches and diarrhoea. For reasons which will become clear, we put him on a Low Allergy Diet. Within seven days of this regime John had been transformed into a new lad. In fact, his mother could not believe the change in him. 'It's like having a new boy in the house!' she said, with a triumphant smile. In stark contrast to his first visit, he sat calmly in the chair for a good twenty minutes as I spoke to his mother about the next stage of his diet. Into the bargain, he was headache-free and his bowels were normal.

John was put on the Low Allergy Diet because of the pioneering work carried out by Professor John Soothill and colleagues at the Great Ormond Street Children's Hospital in London. They found that many children with migraine became headache-free on a diet. They also noticed, to their surprise, that children who had migraine *and* behavioural problems also reported an improvement in behaviour, and not just a reduction of headache, when they were on the diet. This prompted the professor to investigate the role of food intolerance in hyperactivity. To this end he took a group of seventy-six hyperactive children and put them on the diet. Twenty-one improved, an interesting if somewhat teasing result.

This study was followed by another, in which 116 of 185 hyperactive children improved on the diet. Now we are getting somewhere — this is indeed an impressive figure. Think of all the suffering that could be avoided in these young lives by simply sorting out their diets! It should be said that some 27 per cent of the children reported a complete resolution of symptoms. The other children were not necessarily 'completely cured', but they were very much better than before the diet. This is important. We are not saying that food intolerance is the only factor involved in hyperactivity, but it is in some cases. Sorting out the diets of children with hyperactivity will, in many cases, help them overcome their handicap. For full instructions on the Low Allergy Diet see chapter 17.

There are other treatment options for those who do not respond to dietary manipulations. These include behavioural therapy with or without medication. The medication is based on amphetamine, with all of its attendant problems, and is therefore not prescribed lightly.

Could it be anything else?

It is important to distinguish hyperactivity from other conditions with which it may share some features. Depression and anxiety, for example, can occur in children, and will easily affect their behaviour and learning. The other main diagnosis which may need to be considered is that of Conduct Disorder, a rather euphemistic term for various degrees of delinquency! Take the Duke of Burgundy, for example, the grandson of Louis XIV of France. He was described by his guardians in less than glowing terms. 'Monsignor', they said, 'was born with a disposition which made one tremble.' He was said to be so passionate that he would break the clocks when they struck the hour which summoned him to some unwelcome duty, and fly off into the wildest rage at the rain which hindered his pleasure. Resistance would make him perfectly furious. He was intensely obstinate, and desperately fond of good eating and games. It was dangerous to play with him, for he could not endure to be beaten. He was disposed to be cruel, and he looked upon the rest of mankind as an inferior race with which he had nothing in common. Louis was concerned. After all, this young man was successor to the throne! So, in 1689, the king appointed a 'Preceptor of the Duke of Burgundy'. Thus it was that the good Bishop Fénelon was entrusted with the unenviable task of taming 'the wild boy'. With gentle and firm love, it is recorded in history, and over a relatively short period of time, Fénelon succeeded in his task. This we can see from the following description of the lad after Fénelon's influence had an effect: 'The marvel is that, in so short a time, devotion and grace should have made an altogether new being of him and changed so many redoubtable faults into the entirely opposite virtues.' Quite clearly, the duke was in need not of a diet but of loving discipline!

12.II Allergy and the Brain: Migraine and Other Headaches

Headache

Headaches are extremely common in the general population, with up to 90 per cent of adults admitting to at least one headache in the previous twelve months. The vast majority of these are related to stress and fatigue. As such, we refer to them as tension headaches, and we should consider them almost as a 'normal' response to stress. In this chapter, however, I wish to deal specifically with a very different kind of headache, migraine.

CASE HISTORY

Louise was a student who was looking forward to starting at university in the autumn. She suffered from severe headaches throughout her five years at secondary school, and was hoping to study for her degree without the impediment of frequent illness. She experienced her first real attack of headache just a few months after her first menstrual period, and she has had regular attacks ever since.

The headaches were erratic, but always followed the same course. The warning sign was invariably a blurring of vision — she had come to recognise and dread it as the first symptom of an attack. During this phase she would notice that parts of a page would disappear from sight, or that sequences of numbers would appear incomplete. Thus, if she wanted to phone the doctor, she was unable to read the entry in the directory and had to rely on someone else to do it for her. On occasion, these patches of missing vision would progress to total blindness. She also had other frightening symptoms, such as slurred speech and a tingling sensation in her right arm. Within thirty minutes her headache would start. This she described as a searing pain through one temple 'like someone hammering a nail into my brain'.

The headache was always accompanied by nausea and vomiting. During an attack she would withdraw into a darkened room where, she hoped, she could fall asleep in undisturbed silence. This would be her only relief, and she knew that she would feel much better, if a little sore and tired, when she woke. Sometimes, however, the headache would persist for a second day. As far as she knew, the only thing that would trigger an attack was the smell of wet varnish. There was no link between attacks and her menstrual cycle, nor was there any particular food that she knew to avoid. Attacks were random, paying no respect to her social promises or commitments. Indeed, she was so often incapacitated that she hardly ever committed herself to a meeting, nor even to a date. She preferred to live hour by hour: 'If it happens it happens, and if it doesn't, too bad.' Louise has **migraine**.

What is migraine?

Migraine is a paroxysmal headache: it comes and goes in bursts. The headache itself may or may not be preceded by warning signals. These are non-painful experiences related to alterations in vision and the other senses, and we refer to them collectively as the migraine 'aura'. Migraine *with an aura* is called 'classical migraine', and *without an aura* is called 'common migraine' — the latter being twice as common as the former. In textbook descriptions, the migraine aura is said to start with a spot or 'spots in front of the eyes'. These are small to start with, and gradually enlarge. The edges of spreading spots often tingle or sparkle with bright colourful lights. They frequently assume a zigzag appearance as they move across the field of vision. As they enlarge, they leave behind potholes of blurred vision or even no vision, i.e. blind spots. Very rarely, the whole vision is lost during an attack.

Another well-known symptom is altered sensations on the skin. Tingling, pins and needles or numbness often affect the hands, forearms and face — the upper lip being a particularly favoured site. Other strange phenomena may also occur, such as hallucinations or disorientation in time and space. The former consist of a very real sense of having heard or smelt something that no one else can hear or smell. The disoriented patients may feel lost in their own homes.

The headache itself is said to start in the temple area, from where it gradually spreads to cover one side of the head. Indeed, this is why it is called migraine — a word derived from he*micran*ia (half-head). In practice, however, the headache may affect both sides of the head, or may alternate between one side and the other. The pain builds up, over thirty minutes or so, in a throbbing crescendo. Patients seek out quiet and dark places where they can lie down. Light and noise are unbearable to them, and they know that sleep is their only real hope of relief. Many patients feel much better after a sleep and carry on with their lives. For others, however, the headache may last a lot longer, sometimes extending to two or three days.

Once the attack is over, patients feel perfectly well, and may remain so for weeks on end, until the next attack. The frequency of attacks varies enormously between one migraineur and the next. Most migraineurs get one or two attacks per month; some will get away with only one or two attacks in a lifetime; and others get two or three attacks per week. Think about that: several attacks each week which may persist for one or two days at a time! Life for these unfortunates is one continuous headache.

It will serve our purpose well to spend just a little more time on this. Classical migraine, as we have seen, starts with an aura and proceeds to a throbbing headache. This reflects the underlying nature of migraine — it is a 'vascular (blood vessel) headache'. This is what happens. Firstly, of course, something sparks off the attack (and we will address the triggers presently). The blood vessels respond to the trigger by constricting — they shut down — and, in so doing, greatly reduce the amount of blood getting through to the brain. The regions of the brain that are thus deprived of blood kick up a racket. They misfire, sending off all sorts of nervous messages.

The visual disturbances are a good example of this. Light enters the eyeball and is translated into tiny electrical impulses on the retina. These travel along the optic pathway to be projected onto a large full-colour screen at the back of the brain, the occipital cortex. Imagine what would happen if the cortex started to misfire. Areas of the screen would start to flash and sparkle. Further loss of function would lead to areas of visual loss; and a complete power failure, so to speak, would result in an entirely blank screen, blindness.

Hallucinations of smell and hearing simply reflect the very same events taking place in other parts of the brain, the olfactory and auditory cortices. Likewise, the pins and needles, numbness, slurred speech and so on all reflect the same basic problem, *vasoconstriction*. After thirty minutes of vasoconstriction, we get an equal and opposite response, *vasodilatation*. The blood vessels dilate and throb with each and every beat of the heart. Blood vessels in the brain are tender, sensitive structures; so they hurt when they are stretched. That's why migraine is characterised by severe pounding headaches. Common migraine is the *very same headache* without the aura. In other words, there is no significant vasoconstriction, only vasodilatation.

Who gets it?

Ten per cent of the population suffers from migraine. The first migraine attack often occurs in childhood, just after puberty, in the teenage years or in early adulthood. Although it is possible, the first attack is less commonly seen in later decades — with the exception, perhaps, of women who are going through the menopause. Migraine affects women twice as often as men.

Will they grow out of it?

By definition, migraine is a paroxysmal disorder — it recurs at various intervals throughout life. Whereas some of us might have one attack in our lifetime, others are plagued with constant headache. In general, attacks tend to be less frequent and less severe as we approach pensionable age. There are two reasons for this: one of them flattering, the other less so. Firstly, being older and wiser, and more relaxed in retirement, we are less prone to many of the triggers of migraine. Secondly, and perhaps more importantly, our blood vessels get thick and less flexible — hence they cannot bounce around (throb) as they used to.

What causes it?

We don't know the cause of migraine, but once again, this is a condition that runs in families. Up to 90 per cent of patients with classical migraine have a family member who is affected, or has been at some stage. Recent research has identified a gene which is thought to be linked to one form of migraine, the 'paralysing' hemiplegic migraine.

There are several widely recognised migraine triggers, including:

- missing a meal
- excitement
- bright lights
- strong smells
- grinding or clenching the teeth
- minor trauma to the head (heading a football)
- too much sleep (which may explain some 'weekend headaches')
- too little sleep
- too much work
- some medicines, such as the oral contraceptive pill and vasodilators
- menstruation (conversely, migraine often improves in pregnancy!)
- and certain foods

The food and smell triggers are of particular interest to the allergist.

Food intolerance: *a driving force in migraine*

Virtually all migraineurs will have heard about chocolate, cheese, caffeine, citrus fruit and alcohol as known migraine triggers. These foods have one thing in common: they all contain natural substances that exert a direct effect on blood vessels. In other words, these are pharmacologically active foods, they act like drugs, particularly in those who are sensitive to their effects. These sensitive patients may be lacking in an enzyme which would normally deal with the active ingredients. Thus, avoiding the food brings about relief. Some of you will have discovered this for yourselves, but many others will testify to the fact that you still get migraine attacks even though you studiously avoid these foods. Don't despair, there is still much hope for you. Read on.

In 1983 a landmark paper was published in the *Lancet*, in which it was shown that 93 per cent of eighty-eight children with severe and frequent migraine found relief on a Low Allergy Diet. Furthermore, forty of these children were subsequently able to tell which foods gave them a migraine and which ones did not, even though the food was disguised in lentil soup — in other words they were 'blind' to the food being challenged. A similar study carried out in adults gave equally impressive results, in that 85 per cent of patients found relief from migraine whilst on an exclusion diet.* This was in spite of the fact that these patients had, on average, a twenty-year history of severe frequent headache. Between them, they consumed an average of 115 painkillers per month before the diet; this figure plummeted to less than 1 after the diet!

The strong impression that food intolerance is a significant driving force in many cases of migraine has been confirmed time and again by those of us who work in the field. Consider Louise, for instance. We put her on a Low Allergy Diet, and she quickly became headache-free. Not only that, but she felt better than she had done for ages. Having thus satisfied herself that food was an important factor in her migraine, she proceeded to the next stage in the dietary investigation: the sequential reintroduction of foods. Over the following month, as she tested her staple foods one by one, she discovered that wheat and rye could both induce migraine attacks. Other foods could be eaten freely.

Louise now had a choice. She could (i) avoid these foods in the long term, or (ii) go for a course of desensitisation. The latter course of action, if successful, would allow her to eat her problem foods without the migraine penalty. However, she was rather pleased with the fact that she had lost her excess weight on the diet, and she wanted to keep it that way. She feared that desensitisation would allow her to eat wheat, and that she would put the weight back on! She opted for avoidance, and was now confident of being able to study without the worry of another migraine around the corner.

Chemical sensitivity: another driving force in migraine
It is well accepted in medical circles that strong smells can trigger a migraine attack. Like the pharmacologically active foods referred to above, some chemicals have a direct effect on blood vessels, making them dilate, and this is thought to be the mechanism of at least some of these chemical reactions. It is also possible that the stimulus of the olfactory (smell) nerve itself is the important trigger. But I would like to draw your attention to another possibility: some people are very sensitive to environmental chemicals in much the same way that others are allergic to pollen, or intolerant to food.

---

*As an interesting aside, fifteen of these patients — who were known to have high blood pressure (diastolic ≥100 mm Hg) — returned to normal blood pressure (diastolic ≤90 mm Hg) whilst on the diet.

One such patient was Angela, a 35-year-old 'working mother' of two, who had frequent migraine attacks. Significantly, she was never really clear of symptoms between attacks. The headache would abate, sure, but she was left with many other symptoms, namely a permanent feeling of nausea, bloating of the stomach, and generalised aches and pains in her muscles. Being a mother in such circumstances was hard enough, and she feared that the time had finally come to give up her job. She just couldn't cope any more. As I delved into the symptoms in some detail, Angela revealed an important clue. Within seconds of sitting into a new car her vision would blur, her nausea would worsen and her stomach would go into cramps. The old familiar headache would start half an hour later. The smell of new cars gave her migraine! Angela was advised to rid her home of all chemical smells, including deodorants, air fresheners, perfumes, aftershave, polish, etc. Her symptoms were greatly reduced within a fortnight, suggesting that she was indeed a 'chemically sensitive' individual (see chapter 15).

Are there any complications?

Frequent migraine is a very disabling condition which seriously affects the quality of life of some patients. Other complications which may occur, albeit rarely, include the following:

- Very rarely the migraine is continuous (days or weeks on end) and eventually requires hospital treatment. This is called 'status migrainosus'.
- Epileptic attacks can occur at the height of the migraine attack. This is thought to result from prolonged oxygen lack in the brain.
- Mild one-sided weakness is common during a migraine attack. However, some patients experience a more profound loss of power, a partial paralysis. This is called hemiplegic migraine.
- In *very rare* cases, the vasoconstriction behind the loss of power has been extreme and prolonged, resulting in permanent nerve damage in the brain. Permanent loss of vision and permanent loss of power have occurred. It must be stressed that this is extremely rare. Statistically, you have a far greater chance of winning the Lotto twice than ending up with permanent damage.

What can we do about it?

- Avoid the known triggers listed above.
- Avoid pharmacologically active foods, such as *alcohol, chocolate, liver, pickled herring, cured meats, citrus fruit, caffeine and cheese.*
- Take medicines at the onset of an attack to abort it, or at least lessen its severity. Simple aspirin is often as good as anything else. If this fails to relieve the attack, talk to your doctor about using something else. There are several courses of action to choose from.
- Take medicines to prevent attacks, or at least lessen their frequency. Discuss this option with your doctor. Again, there are several options to choose from.
- Check out your 'allergies'.
  1. Go through the Low Allergy Diet outlined in chapter 17. Warning: if you have ever suffered a complete loss of vision during an attack, or if you have ever lost the power of an arm or a leg during an attack, do not diet without consulting an allergy doctor first!
  2. Consider a 'chemical holiday', particularly if you have other symptoms of chemical sensitivity (see chapter 15).

Could it be anything else?

We must remember that there are many other kinds of headache arising from diverse causes. Thus, headache may be caused by:

- Tension
  This is by far the commonest cause of the affliction. These headaches are often felt on the top of the head, or as a tight band around the head. They are present 'most of the day on most days' and they are associated with anxiety. They often get worse in the evenings.
- Eye problems
  Everyone is familiar with the notion that eye strain can cause headache. It is wise therefore to get your eyesight checked to make sure that you don't need glasses. The optician will also screen your eyes for glaucoma, for it too can cause headache.
- Arthritis in the neck
  The nerves which supply sensation to the scalp must pass through rather narrow gaps between the bones in the neck before they eventually feed into the brain. If these gaps are affected by arthritis the available space will be even narrower

than usual and the nerve will get pinched. The brain will think that there is a problem 'somewhere in the scalp', and the patient will interpret this message as a headache. This is particularly important in the elderly. Physiotherapy often provides relief.

- Sinus trouble
  The sinuses are often blamed for headache. However, other signs of sinus disease, such as swelling, tenderness or X-ray evidence, should be present to confirm the diagnosis.
- TMJ problems
  The TMJ (tempero-mandibular joint) is the joint between your jawbone and your skull. It sits just in front of the ear on each side. Between the TMJ and the ear there lies a bundle of nerves and blood vessels. If the joint is not properly aligned it may put pressure on these sensitive structures and cause headache.
- Sex
  Two kinds of headache may occur during or after sexual intercourse. The first builds gradually during foreplay and arousal, and is thought to come from tension in the neck and scalp muscles. The second is an explosive type of headache which occurs at orgasm. The explosion of pain may be so severe that a brain haemorrhage is suspected. Both of these are more common in men, and tend to lessen with the passage of time.
- Head injuries
  Serious head injuries sometimes leave a patient with chronic headaches. The full 'Post-Concussion Syndrome', as it is called, consists of headaches, dizziness, impaired concentration, and irritability of mood. Headaches may also follow relatively minor head injury.
- Diseases of the skull
  Uncommon diseases, such as Paget's disease of the bones, or the even less common deposits of cancer in the bone of the skull, may cause headache.
- Other diseases
  Headache is a frequent companion of many disease states. However, in these cases other symptoms will be prominent, and should draw attention to the underlying problem. One important exception is the headache of cranial arteritis (an inflammation in the arteries that feed the head), but even

here the headache is sufficiently characteristic in nature to alert the doctor to the true cause.

- Brain tumours
  The one we all dread, but this is in fact a very rare cause of chronic headache. There is no connection between migraine and brain tumours or haemorrhages.

12.III Allergy and the Brain: Fatigue

Fatigue is a very common complaint, with up to 20 per cent of men and 30 per cent of women admitting to feeling excessively tired at any one point in time. Most of this fatigue, like the tension headache of chapter 12.II, is related to psychosocial stress; and most of us recover our energies, without help, once the stress has passed. Thus, it is only those who find it difficult or impossible to shake off their fatigue who are likely to visit a doctor. Doctors, for their part, will say that fatigue is one of the most common complaints they are called upon to treat. It is also one of the most difficult.

Reassuringly, only 5 per cent of fatigued patients turn out to have something 'physically' wrong, such as an underactive thyroid gland or a low blood count. Conversely, 70 per cent have an underlying depressive illness or anxiety state. In spite of the social taboo which attends these conditions, they are, in fact, very positive diagnoses. They are made on the grounds of a clinical history replete with other symptoms of depression or anxiety; and, most importantly, they facilitate appropriate and effective treatments for the patient. Thus, we can understand the nature of fatigue in 75 per cent of all cases, and the future is bright for many of these.

We must now consider the remaining 25 per cent of patients whose fatigue defies explanation. These have been through the usual mill of investigation: physical examination is normal, the blood tests draw a blank, and the psychiatrist gives a clean bill of mental health. 'Well then, doctor, why on earth am I feeling so tired all the time?' This patient is now frustrated with his condition, and dissatisfied with his physician. But doctors are human, they are equally frustrated, and will often confess that they, too, are dissatisfied with the quality of care they deliver to the fatigued. In trying to solve the problem, a brave doctor might venture further: 'You know, Mr Jones, sometimes fatigue is the only symptom of depression.' 'That's a load of twaddle, doctor!' comes the sharp and angry reply, 'Surely I would know whether I was depressed or not?'

The doctor's suggestion, however, is not all twaddle. Patients do *not* always know when they are depressed! And fatigue *is* sometimes the covert forerunner of depression. In these cases, and given sufficient time, the other features of depression will eventually become clear. But this 'hidden depression' should not be confused with the depression that so often afflicts the chronically ill. Bear in mind that up to 65 per cent of patients with chronic illness *will* suffer from reactive depression or anxiety at some stage during their illness, whatever the illness. The fatigue states are no exception to this, and studies repeatedly show that patients with chronic unexplained fatigue frequently become depressed in the course of their illness — *because of their illness*. Notwithstanding, many patients testify that they have been unfairly dismissed as being 'just stressed out' or 'depressed', when they know well they are not, and when the passage of time proves them right.

As you can see, we are dealing with a very complex problem, but the bottom line is stark and simple: we have amongst us a group of patients who suffer from chronic debilitating fatigue of unknown origin. For our part, as doctors and carers, we must learn to sit silently and respectfully with what we cannot yet understand. Above all, we must resist the indefensible practice of assigning these patients to a diagnostic dumping ground of convenience. It is simply not good enough — and it is certainly not good medicine — to say that 'We can find nothing wrong so it *must* be in your head.'

At the end of the day, many of these patients will turn out to have idiopathic (we-don't-know-the-cause) fatigue, and some will eventually receive a diagnosis of Chronic Fatigue Syndrome (CFS). These rank amidst the most challenging of all medical disorders — but such a confession does not constitute a veiled surrender. On the contrary, we must repudiate the general notion that 'nothing can be done' for the fatigued patient. Why? Because, in many cases, it simply isn't true! Furthermore, and I can promise you this, some will find lasting relief in this chapter.

CASE HISTORY

Dorothy was a secretary in her local hospital. She was suffering from chronic fatigue, and found it increasingly difficult to cope. She described herself as 'not the type that gives in easily', and she proved her assertion by saving every ounce of energy for work. However, there was a price to pay for such perseverance and courage: she had no energy left for anything else. At first, she gave up her sporting activities, and then other aspects of her social life. She thought that cutting back in this manner would help her to recover. It didn't. Her world thus contracted to two activities, work and sleep. She collapsed into bed every evening as soon as she returned from work, and spent whole weekends in bed, trying to recuperate some energy for the week ahead. Eventually, she could cope no more.

The doctor examined her, and ran a series of blood tests. He also spent some considerable time going into the details of Dorothy's personal life. He was, of course, looking for signs of depression, but he found none. Dorothy loved her work. She also loved a young man to whom she was engaged, and the relationship seemed harmonious enough. The doctor also took note of other symptoms, such as headaches, generalised aches and pains, and recurrent sore throats. He knew his patient of old, and confirmed that she was indeed a hardy type who seldom called on his services. He flicked through her case notes and read the last entry.

It was nine months ago, and he remembered it well. Her mother had phoned in a bit of a panic, and asked him to come urgently to the house. Dorothy was very ill indeed, there was no doubt. She was in bed with fever, headache, drenching sweats, and nausea. What really worried him, however, was the incessant vomiting and stiff neck. He admitted her to hospital where she was treated for meningitis, and where, thankfully, she made an excellent recovery — or, at least, he thought she had. 'What happened after that, Dorothy?' the doctor enquired. 'Well,' she said, 'I've never been right since then, and if you ask me, that's when all my trouble started.'

The doctor was now in a position to offer her a tentative diagnosis. He would have to keep an open mind, of course, but until something shows up to prove otherwise, Dorothy is suffering from a **Chronic Fatigue Syndrome.***

---

*CFS has been called by many other names, including myalgic encephalomyelitis (ME), Postviral Fatigue Syndrome (PVFS), Royal Free disease, Icelandic disease, etc. None of these names is entirely satisfactory. They reflect our attempts to guess the underlying cause, or the names of places in which significant and well-documented epidemics have occurred.

What is Chronic Fatigue Syndrome?

Chronic Fatigue Syndrome is characterised by a fatigue which cannot be explained by physical or psychiatric means, and which . . .

1. is of new or definite onset
2. is persistent or relapsing
3. has been present for at least six months
4. is not due to 'overdoing it'
5. is not substantially relieved by rest
6. results in a substantial reduction in previous levels of
   - occupational activity
   and/or
   - social activity
   and/or
   - personal activity
   and/or
   - educational activity

In addition, there must also be four or more of the following symptoms:

1. recurrent sore throats
2. tender glands in the neck or under the arms
3. muscle pains
4. joint pain
5. headaches
6. unrefreshing sleep
7. difficulty recovering from exertion

It stands to reason that these symptoms, like the fatigue they accompany, should also be of new onset. Thus the joint pains of pre-existing arthritis, or the headache of a patient with a history of migraine, should not count towards a diagnosis of CFS. However, if the joint pains or headache, etc., are of new severity or quality then they are taken into account. Similarly, we do not diagnose CFS in patients who have . . .

1. other medical explanations of fatigue, such as a low blood count, unresolved hepatitis, etc.
2. a past or current diagnosis of psychotic depression, manic depression, schizophrenia, delusional disorders, dementia, anorexia nervosa or bulimia nervosa
3. a history of alcohol or substance abuse two years prior to onset of their fatigue, or at any other time thereafter
4. a problem with severe obesity

Before the discerning reader objects, let me acknowledge that these diagnostic criteria are fallible. Who, for example, is to say that one patient does not have CFS because they have been ill for just under six months, and that another does because they are ill for six months and a day? Similarly, we acknowledge from the outset that this arbitrary definition will exclude those who have a less severe or less typical form of chronic fatigue. Furthermore, patients with psychiatric disorders are not immune from allergies, infections, cancer or any other disease. Who, then, can deny them the 'right' to develop a Chronic Fatigue Syndrome? Notwithstanding, these criteria do serve a very important purpose. They allow us to identify, with at least some degree of international consistency, a group of patients whose lives are significantly affected by debilitating fatigue. It is this group which offers our research efforts the best chance of a breakthrough. If we can understand their condition, we will begin to understand the less severe forms of fatigue as well.

Idiopathic chronic fatigue
Patients whose fatigue cannot be explained, but who do not ful-fil all of the diagnostic criteria for CFS, are said to suffer from idiopathic fatigue. But, as we have said, this is an arbitrary decision. Idiopathic fatigue is no less debilitating than the fatigue of a full-blown CFS.

Who gets it?

Anyone can get CFS, although we do not like to diagnose it in very young children. My oldest patient was an 83-year-old woman, my youngest a nine-year-old boy, both of whom recovered. It occurs most commonly in women in the second and third decades of life. Contrary to popular opinion, CFS is not the preserve of the young and upwardly mobile. Thus, the derogatory term 'yuppie flu' should be regarded as tabloid trash. Nor is it the preserve of any particular social class or race. Cases have occurred throughout the world, and I am happy to say that this is reflected in the international scientific community: doctors and scientists from all over the world meet on a regular basis to exchange information and to discuss avenues of research.

Will they grow out of it?

A great number of patients recover completely, and return to full and active lives. Some of these now run their own business, others pursue a trade or profession, and some even play competitive sports at national and international level. Having said that, and although the average duration of illness is said to be three to six years, a minority remain ill for years on end.

What causes it?

We do not know the cause of CFS; and although 80 per cent of cases, like Dorothy's above, start in the immediate aftermath of a viral infection, we have so far failed to understand the mechanism. There is an increasing body of evidence which suggests that the fundamental problem lies in the way the brain works. Thus, several hormonal pathways in the brain are known to malfunction in CFS. Furthermore, the pattern of malfunction is quite different from what one sees in the depressed brain or in the anxious brain — more evidence that CFS is nòt 'just another form of depression'.

Another significant clue is that up to 50 per cent of patients with CFS have a history of allergic disorders, such as hay fever, asthma, eczema or urticaria. That's a lot more than one would expect from the general population. Similarly, and even more significantly, up to 70 per cent of CFS patients currently show activation of their eosinophils — a very important cell in allergic disease (hence the inclusion of a chapter on CFS in a book dealing with allergies). However, as interesting as they are, these abnormalities — hormonal, brain and immune — are still only scattered pieces of the jigsaw. We have a long way to go before we understand the fatigue states.

Are there any complications?

CFS is, by definition, a debilitating illness. Affected patients may have to put their lives on hold. It would be impossible for me to describe their frustration, so I won't even try. However, think about the strain their illness brings to bear on their close relationships, their career aspirations, their finances, and, eventually, their mental health. It is not surprising that so many become depressed as a result — indeed, sometimes to the point of suicidal thought. Treating the depression is, of course, helpful. But treating the depression does not remove the fatigue.

What can we do about it?

I want to highlight the 'allergic' aspects of CFS, and I will therefore concentrate on these. The full management plan for patients with CFS is beyond the scope of this text, but briefly summarised:

1. Secure the diagnosis with your doctor. This will involve a careful clinical history, a thorough physical examination, and a few basic blood tests to rule out other disorders.
2. Pay a great deal of attention to the sleep pattern. Establish a regular night's sleep by whatever means necessary. This will often require the use of medication — *but not the use of sleeping tablets.* Specifically, correct insomnia, or excessive sleeping, or abnormal sleeping hours — all of which occur regularly in CFS.
3. Consider the use of nutritional supplements, but get expert advice on this.
4. Consider the use of intramuscular magnesium injections; again get expert advice.
5. Consider the use of antidepressants, even if there is no evidence of overt depression. The chemical pathways in the brain which are responsible for mood are also responsible for energy levels and sleep patterns. Thus, a drug which affects mood will also affect energy levels.
6. Consider a graduated exercise programme, and I emphasise *graduated.* We know that 'too much too soon' will bring on a relapse. We also know that a properly conducted exercise programme is of great benefit.
7. Avoid alcohol, caffeine, nicotine and refined sugars — they only make matters worse.
8. Check out your diet for food intolerance!

Food intolerance: an unrecognised cause of chronic fatigue

Brenda was a forty-year-old housewife with all the symptoms of a Chronic Fatigue Syndrome. Her trouble started, two years ago, with a viral infection of the thyroid gland. She was perfectly well before this, but never right since. In particular, she complained of bouts of extreme fatigue, recurrent sore throats, pains in the arms and legs, stiffness across the shoulders, swollen glands in her neck, headaches and unrefreshing sleep. She had not been symptom-free for a single day in the past two years. She consulted her doctor frequently, first with one thing and then with another. She found this hard to cope with for, as she said of herself, she took pride in the fact that she hardly ever 'bothered the doctor'.

Everything was normal on physical examination. The blood tests were also normal; and so, in view of the ongoing symptoms, her doctor referred her to the Allergy Clinic. Brenda went on the Low Allergy Diet and within ten days *all of her symptoms abated*. Two years of abject misery came to an end simply by changing her diet! Subsequent food challenges revealed that she had **multiple food intolerance**. She reacted very badly to wheat, especially, but also to a host of 'otherwise harmless' foods, including bananas, onion, yeast, mushrooms, rice and oats. Because it would have been very difficult to avoid all of these foods, and to prevent the development of other food intolerance, she was offered a course of desensitisation. She has never looked back.

I would also like to introduce you to Gerry. He was a young lad in his early teens who complained of constant fatigue. His mother told me that he had never really recovered from a glandular fever three years previously. She described him as lethargic, always sitting down, with no real energy or interest in anything. For his part, Gerry also complained of frequent bellyaches, recurrent sore throats, and dizzy spells. He too was placed on the Low Allergy Diet, and he too lost all of his symptoms. He reacted badly to wheat, rye and oats — all gluten-containing foods. He had a biopsy test to exclude coeliac disease (see p. 141), and this was negative. We can safely say, therefore, that Gerry had a post-glandular fever fatigue prolonged by food intolerance — in his case, non-coeliac gluten intolerance.

In both of these cases there is a clear history of viral onset. One had a thyroid infection; the other a glandular fever. In each case, the patient slid imperceptibly from a state of viral infection into one of food intolerance. Patients have been known to develop IgE allergies, such as hay fever and asthma, in the wake of viral infection; but the development of food intolerance under similar circumstances has received less attention. This is a pity because, as these cases so clearly demonstrate, postviral food intolerance can cause years of suffering.

Could it be anything else?

CFS is a diagnosis of exclusion — it should be entertained only after a thorough medical assessment has failed to identify a known cause of fatigue. Such an assessment should also include a sympathetic evaluation of the patient's mental state. This is particularly important, for stress and depression are the most common causes of fatigue, and we should not underestimate the prominence that fatigue may assume in these circumstances.

Depression: moody tiredness

Four years ago Paddy came down with the flu. He described himself as 'unwell ever since'. He complained of fatigue, sore muscles and bones, and a disturbed sleep pattern. So far, his symptoms could have been considered 'a possible case of CFS', and this was the reason for his referral. However, as we delved a little further into his symptoms, Paddy gave a very clear picture of depression, and it became obvious that he was not suffering from a Postviral Fatigue Syndrome. His tiredness was described as 'a moody tiredness, a weariness — like a heavy weight holding me down'. He had lost interest in his job, he didn't feel like socialising, and he avoided situations that he had relished heretofore. He was socially withdrawn, and he had lost all sense of pleasure in life. Finally, his sleep disruption was classical of depression: he woke every morning at 4 a.m., and try as he might, he could not get back to sleep again.

We spoke at length about his depression, but we could not find an obvious cause for it. He was happily married with a few healthy kids, his business ventures were going well, he had no financial difficulties and there were no recent stresses. In spite of all that, Paddy was depressed, and quite considerably so. His fatigue was simply part and parcel of that. We should now look again at Paddy's original flu. He clearly thought it was responsible for his plight. However, we have just said that he was *not* suffering from a Postviral Fatigue Syndrome. What role, then, did the virus play in all of this? The answer is quite simple: viral infections not only induce fatigue states, they can give rise to depression.

Anxiety: restless tiredness

Jenny was convinced that she had multiple food allergies. She was sure that these were the cause of her chronic fatigue. She thought, for example, that onions gave her a bloated tummy, that yeast and bread gave her a rapid heartbeat, and that beef gave her diarrhoea and a jittery feeling in the pit of her stomach. However, she would still experience these symptoms when she avoided (what she thought were) her troublesome foods. That's why she thought that she had other food allergies not yet discovered.

But her symptoms were of interest in their own right. Look at them for a moment apart from the foods which were said to cause them. She was tired all the time, she had bouts of diarrhoea and a bloated abdomen, her heart was beating too fast, and she felt jittery in the pit of her stomach. These are physical symptoms of anxiety, and they call for further exploration. 'Well, yes,' she confessed, 'I am a bit of a worrier.' Jenny frequently stayed awake for hours at night thinking about the events of the day, worrying about her children, and planning her chores for the morning. She also described having to live through many days with 'a strange feeling of something bad about to happen'. Nothing particularly bad ever did happen, but Jenny was unable to calm her mind with such reassuring thoughts. She had an *anxiety disorder*, and her fatigue was just a manifestation of that.

Jenny was encouraged to eat all foods, even those she thought were making her ill. Meanwhile she was given some medical treatment for her anxiety. She improved greatly over the following few months.

Also consider these

- Narcolepsy: sleepy tiredness
  Mary Beth came to the clinic with her mother. Tiredness had been her constant unwelcome companion throughout all of her secondary school years. She was now about to sit her final exams, but she feared that she would fail because she had missed so much study. Her classmates had nicknamed her 'Dozy', because Mary Beth fell asleep in almost every single class! She also fell asleep at mass, watching TV, in waiting rooms and on buses. In fact, she would fall asleep at the drop of a hat. Furthermore, sometimes she would feel completely paralysed as she woke from sleep — a rather frightening experience for anyone. These symptoms suggested that Mary Beth was suffering from a sleep disorder known as narcolepsy. She was, therefore, admitted to a special sleep disorders unit where the diagnosis was confirmed. She should do well with appropriate treatment.
- Sleep apnoea: snoring tiredness
  Sarah also had a sleep disorder. She first presented to me when she was fifty years old. She complained that she had been dogged with fatigue for all of her adult life. She also had a host of other symptoms, including 'thumping heartbeats', sweats, and swelling of the ankles. She had pains in her arms and legs, bloating of the abdomen, and constipation.

What was of particular interest, however, was the fact that she, too, could fall asleep anywhere. She had more control over this than Mary Beth, but it was a problem nevertheless. When questioned further, she admitted to snoring during her sleep. She had never heard it herself, of course, but she snored so loudly that her friends would now refuse to share a bedroom with her on holidays! 'They tell me I snore like a sawmill!' she said. Moreover, on more than one occasion she scared the living daylights out of her room-mates. They would tell her that she suddenly stopped snoring during the night, and that she stopped breathing altogether! The silence seemed to go on for ever, and just as one of them was about to make sure she was still alive, Sarah would give an almighty snort, and settle down into her snoring routine again.

Sleep studies confirmed that Sarah had **sleep apnoea** — a sleep disorder related to snoring. The airway is partially blocked by 'floppy' soft tissues in the nose and throat. These tissues flap against each other when air is passing through the airway, and the flapping gives rise to the snore. During deep sleep, the airway collapses completely — hence the prolonged silence described above. The problem here is that air is no longer getting into the lungs. The unconscious breathing drive is not strong enough to overcome the obstruction, so a panic message is sent to the brain. The brain responds by waking up for a microsecond — just long enough to initiate a more 'conscious' breathing drive, but not long enough for the patient to remember. The patient then snorts loudly in taking the 'conscious' breath. However, the sleep architecture is seriously disrupted in the process, and the end result is non-restorative sleep. Treatments are available and they are quite effective.

- Caffeine: drugged tiredness*
Too much caffeine can cause fatigue! 'But I thought caffeine was a stimulant,' you may say — and it is. However, when taken in excess it gives rise to fatigue, insomnia, 'restless legs' (in bed at night), a racing heart, shakes, headaches and mood changes.

- Hypoglycaemia*
This is a condition in which blood sugar levels blow around like a kite in the wind. It is related to a diet containing too many sweet things — foods which the patient paradoxically craves.

---

*These conditions have been addressed in *Feeling Tired All the Time*.

- Hyperventilation*
  This is the subconscious habit of overbreathing, and is frequently related to underlying stress. The chemical changes which ensue in the blood are responsible for the fatigue.
- Nutritional insufficiency*
  Adequate supplies of vitamins and minerals are essential to health and energy. Outright nutritional deficiencies are relatively rare in our society, but that does not necessarily mean that we are all enjoying states of optimum nutrition.
- Parasite infection*
  Listed here because parasites are not always 'rowdy', they may be silently living in the gut. Furthermore, they may elude our first attempts to find them. Modern techniques are improving our detection rate.
- Gut fermentation
  See chapter 14.
- Chemical sensitivity
  See chapter 15.

---

*These conditions have been addressed in *Feeling Tired All the Time*.

13 Allergy and Rheumatism

There are at least 100 different ways in which joints and their surrounding tissues can be affected by disease. We refer to these collectively as rheumatic disorders. This rather imprecise terminology includes conditions which, on the face of it, have nothing much in common: they have many different causes and they give rise to very different symptoms. Thus, lumbago and gout, tennis elbow and frozen shoulder, rheumatoid arthritis and spondylitis, are all huddled together under this broad umbrella we call 'rheumatism'. The one thing they do have in common, however, is that they are all characterised by inflammation. Needless to say, it would be impossible to cover all these disorders in a single chapter. My focus is once again restricted to the possible involvement of 'allergy' in rheumatism.

Healthy joints and connective tissue

Joints are specialised structures. They are the interface (articular surface) by which a range of movement may occur between one bone and another. The real wonder of healthy joints is that they allow movement to occur over many years without suffering too much by way of loss or damage. This is possible because the articular surface is so smooth and so well lubricated. Smoothness is provided by a layer of shiny cartilage at the end of each adjoining bone, and lubrication is provided by a special 'oil' we call synovial fluid. Synovial fluid is secreted into the joint by the synovium — the lining of the joint. Strength and stability are afforded to joints by the supportive structures which surround them. These include the joint capsule, several ligaments, and, of course, the muscles which do the moving. In health, we are never really aware of our muscles or joints. But if they should become stiff, painful or swollen they will quickly demand a great deal of attention.

Case history

Lucy was now in her early forties, and she had been troubled by joint pain since her twenties. At first, the 'attacks' of joint pain, as she called them, were few and far between, so she carried on with minimal requirement for painkillers. Of late, however, the pains had become more severe and more consistent. In addition, her joints were swollen and tender, and the pains were disrupting her sleep. She also complained that the 'slight touch' of stiffness which she had learned to live with had become much more bothersome. It took much longer to get out of bed, wash herself and dress. In fact, she now had to set her alarm clock to wake an hour earlier than usual. She was also concerned about her lack of mobility around the office, and the fact that sitting in meetings was now always followed by her joints 'seizing up'. Her doctor carried out a few blood tests, and these confirmed that Lucy was suffering from a flare-up of her **rheumatoid arthritis**.

What is rheumatoid arthritis?

Rheumatoid arthritis is a chronic inflammatory disease of the joints. Specifically, it is the synovium — the special lining of the joints — which is inflamed. This has several effects. In the first place, the synovium itself becomes thickened; secondly, excessive amounts of fluid build up in the joint; and thirdly, the inflammatory cells have a destructive effect on cartilage. Such a joint will be stiff. It will also be swollen (with synovium and fluid) and it will be painful. As the disease progresses, the cartilage suffers further damage, the bone is eroded, the joint becomes clogged with fibrous (scar) tissue, and the soft tissue structures around the joint lose their supportive strength. Eventually, the joint becomes unstable and deformed. In some cases of rheumatoid disease, the inflammatory process affects tissues other than joints. This is not a well-known fact, for we tend to think of arthritis as a disease of the joints only. But the dry eyes of keratoconjunctivitis sicca (see p. 89), for example, are a common finding. So too is anaemia — the result, amongst other things, of defective blood manufacture. Other organs, such as the skin, nerves, blood vessels, heart and lungs, are less commonly inflamed.

The disease usually starts gradually with vague feelings of fatigue and malaise. The first real symptom of joint inflammation is stiffness. Thus, patients often complain of stiffness long before any other symptom, and particularly so in the mornings. Patients will say that it takes them half an hour, or longer, to loosen up after a night's sleep; and they find that sitting for prolonged periods of time has the same stiffening effect. Pain and swelling of the joints become prominent features as the disease progresses. This in turn leads to restriction of movement and loss of muscle power around affected joints.

Rheumatoid arthritis is distinguished from other forms of arthritis on the basis of symptoms. In other words, it is a clinical diagnosis. In particular, the pattern of joint involvement is examined to see whether it fits the diagnosis. Blood tests and X-rays may support the diagnosis, but they are not without their shortcomings. In rheumatoid arthritis:

- Many joints are affected at the same time.
- The small joints of the hands are most commonly affected.
- There is symmetry between affected joints: if one hand is affected so is the other one; if one knee is affected, so is the other one, and so on.
- Joints in the neck are affected in a third of cases, but the rest of the spine is usually not.
- Stiffness is prominent, especially first thing in the morning.
- Other features of rheumatoid disease may be present, such as lumps (nodules) under the skin.
- X-rays may reveal characteristic joint damage (erosions in the bone).
- A positive blood test for 'rheumatoid factor' would support the diagnosis. Rheumatoid factor is an IgM antibody found in the blood of many patients with rheumatoid arthritis. However, it is also found in other immune diseases, and it is not present in all patients with rheumatoid arthritis. Confusing, isn't it? If a given patient has the clinical features of rheumatoid arthritis and a *positive* blood test, we say they have *seropositive* arthritis. If, on the other hand, they have the features of rheumatoid arthritis with a *negative* test, we say they have *seronegative* arthritis.

Who gets it?

One per cent of the adult population have rheumatoid arthritis. Women are three or four times more likely to be affected than men. Although it can start at any time from childhood to old age, it usually starts between the fourth and sixth decades of life. In children (under the age of sixteen years) we call it chronic juvenile arthritis.

Will they grow out of it?

Rheumatoid arthritis is a progressive disease. In most cases the disease follows a fairly constant course, with little by way of fluctuations. Others have intermittent disease. They suffer bouts of arthritis lasting up to a year at a time, and then enjoy several months or years in remission before the next relapse. We can expect 80 per cent of children with the disease to do well, although many will have ongoing problems with relapse and remission, and some will develop a more severe and persistent arthritis.

What causes it?

We don't know the cause of rheumatoid arthritis. However, we suspect a genetic involvement, for many patients with rheumatoid arthritis carry a gene called 'HLA-DR4'. We also have an impression that hormones are important because it occurs much more commonly in women, and it very often improves during pregnancy. Some experts say that a virus could be responsible, and this may be true, but all attempts to identify a culprit have so far failed. Having thus paid homage to established doctrine, I would like to draw your attention to two other possibilities, namely molecular mimicry and food intolerance. Let's take a look at molecular mimicry first. It is, admittedly, a little complicated, but your efforts to grasp these concepts will be richly rewarded!

Molecular mimicry in rheumatoid arthritis

We have just seen that many patients with RA have the HLA-DR4 gene. This genetic molecule is very similar to a molecule found on the 'coat' of a bacterium called proteus. In fact, these molecules are so similar that they are said to *mimic* each other.

Proteus, like any bug, will stimulate the immune system when it tries to infect the body. As we discussed in chapter 2, the immune system responds to the threat of invasion by producing antibodies. These antibodies are specific. They circulate in the blood and will recognise proteus more efficiently next time round. But there is a problem in patients with rheumatoid arthritis: they have a genetic molecule that looks very similar to proteus. The theory of molecular mimicry is based on this similarity.

The antibodies which have been programmed to react against proteus will now react against the HLA-DR4 molecule *in the mistaken belief that it is proteus!* In doing so, the immune system destroys its own joints (and other tissues) — this antibody is a turncoat, it has unwittingly become an 'auto-antibody'.

'Okay, that's interesting,' you may say, 'But why is rheumatoid arthritis more common in women?' Because proteus is a very frequent cause of urinary tract infection, and urinary tract infections are ten times more common in women! It stands to reason, then, that women will have more exposure to proteus; that they will produce more antibodies to fight it; and — if they happen to be HLA-DR4 positive — that they are more likely to start reacting against their own tissues. (We are indebted to Dr Alan Ebringer, of the University of London and Middlesex Hospital, for his pioneering work in this field. His contribution may lead to the development of more effective treatments for rheumatoid arthritis and related disorders.)

Food intolerance in rheumatoid arthritis

Let us now come back to Lucy, the woman who presented to her doctor with a flare-up of arthritis. She was offered 'stronger drugs', but was keen to explore other therapeutic possibilities. She was unhappy with the notion that drugs would only suppress her symptoms, without getting to the root cause of them. She was, therefore, well motivated, and open to the suggestion of dietary intervention. I should also point out, before we proceed, that there were other clues of food intolerance in her history. She complained of bloating of the abdomen, bouts of diarrhoea, abdominal pain, and indigestion — the symptoms of an irritable bowel.

Lucy went on a Low Allergy Diet for fourteen days. When she returned for review she told me proudly that her stomach had settled and, more importantly, that her morning stiffness had disappeared, her sleep was no longer disrupted by joint pain, and her requirement for painkillers was much less than before. We therefore felt justified in pursuing the role of food intolerance in her case. Reintroducing foods one by one, Lucy discovered that her joint pains flared up again whenever she ate banana, chicken, beef, soy bean and wheat. At the time of writing, one year later, she remains free of symptoms — not even the 'slight touch' of stiffness which she had come to accept as normal.

It is important to realise that Lucy's diet was not based on guesswork. On the contrary, it was based on published medical work. For example, in 1981, the *British Medical Journal* published the case of a 38-year-old woman with an eleven-year history of severe rheumatoid disease. She had been treated with all of the usual anti-inflammatory drugs, including aspirin, the non-steroidals and eventually steroids. She was also given gold injections and other very potent immuno-suppressing drugs, but all efforts to contain her symptoms either failed, or had to be withdrawn on account of side effects.

Fortunately, her physician was a bright spark. His curiosity was aroused by the observation that her relatives brought her daily supplies of cheese! When he asked her about it, she happily confessed that she had a passion for cheese, and that she had eaten one pound of this food every day since her early twenties. He invited her to try a dairy exclusion diet on a purely empirical basis, a sort of 'let's-try-it-and-see-what-happens' approach. Within three weeks she began to feel better. Her synovitis and morning stiffness diminished and eventually disappeared altogether. Her case was followed for ten months before it was reported, thus making a placebo (psychological) effect unlikely (see chapter 16). She remained well and fully mobile, apart from when she inadvertently ate dairy produce.

These anecdotes, and others like them, inspired researchers to systematically explore the role of food intolerance in rheumatoid arthritis. On one such occasion, the journal *Clinical Allergy* reported that twenty of twenty-two patients with the disease improved on exclusion diets; and in another study, published in the *Lancet*, thirty-three of forty-five rheumatoid patients described themselves as 'better' or 'much better' after dietary investigation.

There can be little doubt, then, that food intolerance is an important factor in rheumatoid arthritis. However, as discussed in a previous chapter, we do not understand the mechanisms by which food can cause such devastating symptoms. One possibility worth mentioning is the link between food intolerance and molecular mimicry. Drastic changes to the diet, such as occur during dietary investigation for food intolerance, can affect bacterial populations in the gut. Thus, it is conceivable that the diet seriously reduces the numbers of proteus organisms growing in the bowel. If this were so, it could explain why some patients get better during dietary interventions. However, this mechanism could not explain the more straightforward dairy allergy described above. In these cases, it is possible that antibodies bind to food allergens and end up being 'dumped' in the joints. It is also possible that the principle of molecular mimicry will turn out to be applicable to certain foods as well as to bacteria — in other words, that food molecules may also fool the immune system into fighting its own tissues.

Are there any complications?

Progressive disease will lead eventually to joint deformity, and this is what is so disabling. Having said that, the vast majority of patients do quite well. Fifty per cent show little or no disability and 40 per cent show moderate disability. Sadly, 10 per cent of patients with rheumatoid arthritis end up severely disabled. Other complications include the following:

- Osteoporosis (brittle bones) may develop after years of disease. This will happen to any bone which is not called upon to 'stay fit'. The prolonged inactivity enforced on arthritic bones leads to a loss of bone mass. They become brittle as a result, and brittle bones are more easily broken than hard ones.
- Joint infections occur more readily in diseased joints. Suspect this if only one arthritic joint is causing trouble whilst the rest of the joints are 'quiet' — particularly if there is a history of recent infection.
- The drugs used in the treatment of rheumatoid arthritis are not without side effects. However, we must be sensible here. Your doctor will weigh the benefits of treatment against the risk of side effects, and the risk of not treating you. The most potent drugs are also the most likely to cause adverse effects, so these are reserved for patients with more severe disease.

What can we do about it?

1. Learn about the condition, and realise that most patients do very well in the long term.
2. Rest during flare-ups. Sometimes hospital admission is required to ensure that joints are not further stressed by patients having to care for themselves during severe exacerbations. Your doctor may advise that splints be applied to badly inflamed joints for a while.
3. Exercise! But don't put undue stress on the joints. Swimming is excellent for this purpose. When pains are bad, exercise

may be limited to passive movements, i.e. the physiotherapist moves the joints for you. Such exercise is aimed at maintaining a full range of movement in the joints. When you are able for it, the physiotherapist will advise you on muscle strengthening exercises; and later again, on aerobic fitness (within your capabilities).

4. Other physiotherapy treatments which may help include ultrasound, hydrotherapy (exercises in water) and wax baths, to name but a few.

5. Adapt your home to suit your ability. For example, would a second handrail help you up and down the stairs? Would it be easier to get in and out of the bath if you had a simple grip fitted to a wall? Would it be easier to get out of a chair if the seat was a little higher than it is at the moment? An occupational therapist will help you to decide on which practical measures would be of benefit to you.

6. Discuss the use of medicines with your doctor. Simple painkillers are useful in early or mild disease, but they have no effect on the disease itself. Anti-inflammatory drugs, on the other hand, do have an effect on the underlying disease. They also have a painkilling effect. There are numerous drugs to choose from in this category, and you may need to chop and change a bit until you find the one that suits you best. For many patients with rheumatoid arthritis this is all the treatment they will need. Patients who do not respond to anti-inflammatories may be offered the stronger anti-rheumatic drugs, such as gold injections, penicillamine and chloroquine. These will help up to 70 per cent of patients with severe disease, but they are more toxic than the anti-inflammatories.

7. Check out your 'allergies'! Consider the Low Allergy Diet as described in chapter 17. And this advice is not just for the adults with arthritis, it's for the children as well.

Avril was twelve years of age when I first met her. She presented with a two-year history of what her doctors called 'juvenile rheumatoid arthritis'. Her symptoms had started suddenly, and were so severe that she was admitted to hospital for treatment. Since then she has had more or less constant pain in her joints, but she had given up taking her drugs because they gave her a serious bellyache (which turned out to be an ulcer), and besides 'they were no good anyway!' Avril required occasional courses of steroid tablets to control her worst symptoms, and she had consequently put on a lot of weight. It is significant that she also had other allergic complaints, such as a history of asthma, and an Irritable Bowel Syndrome. After a fourteen-day Low Allergy Diet her symptoms had abated. Her stomach troubles settled down, and her joint pains were a lot better. In fact, Avril said that she hadn't felt as well for at least four years. Subsequent food challenges revealed her culprit foods, and a course of desensitisation has enabled her to eat these with impunity, without suffering from the penalty of arthritis.

Could it be anything else?

Rheumatoid arthritis can be a difficult diagnosis to make, particularly in the early days of disease, and when the blood test for rheumatoid factor is negative. Time and space prohibit me from going into all the other possible causes of rheumatism, but I would like to mention something about non-specific joint and muscle pain.

A word about fibromyalgia: 'non-specific rheumatism'

Fionnuala was a 29-year-old housewife who complained of 'general tenderness in the bones'. She was also lacking in energy. Her symptoms had been present since the birth of her third child, a boy now aged five years. Significantly, her sleep was badly disrupted by the new arrival. At first, the pains were affecting only one joint at a time. Then they flitted around from one joint to the next. After some time, and in spite of several visits to the doctor, her symptoms became worse. She was now quite stiff in the mornings, and her muscles were sore to touch. She could not stand being bumped into in a crowd. Nor could she endure being hugged. She was 'sore all over' and, at this stage, quite miserable with the whole affair. She was difficult to diagnose. Her symptoms did not fit a recognised pattern for arthritis and her blood tests were negative. She did, however, fit the diagnosis of **fibromyalgia.**

Fibromyalgia is a disorder of unknown cause affecting up to 4 per cent of the general population. It is more common in women. A large number of other symptoms may be present, including fatigue, morning stiffness, sleep disturbance and headache. Although we do not know what causes the condition, we do suspect that sleep disruption is an important contributing factor, particularly in the early days of onset. Once the condition becomes established it can be difficult to shift, even after a regular sleep pattern is secured.

The fatigue that accompanies fibromyalgia is profound, so much so that it may be confused with the fatigue of Chronic Fatigue Syndrome. Although the symptoms of these two conditions overlap significantly, they are nevertheless separate and distinct clinical entities. Simply put, the dominant symptom in fibromyalgia is pain, whereas in CFS it's fatigue. Fibromyalgia patients will say, 'Get rid of my pain, I can live with the fatigue,' and CFS patients will say, 'Get rid of my fatigue, I can live with the pain.'

Fibromyalgia has one other thing in common with CFS. It, too, is a taboo subject in the minds of many conventional doctors. This is so because fibromyalgia, like CFS, is a clinical diagnosis (made on the grounds of the pattern of symptoms only); and because pain, like fatigue, cannot be measured objectively or confirmed by laboratory tests. Furthermore, depression and anxiety often complicate the clinical picture, and this has led some to suggest that fibromyalgia is really a 'psychogenic rheumatism' — in much the same way that CFS is said to be 'just another form of depression'. However, and for those who will take the time to read them, several studies have established that fibromyalgia and CFS are neither psychosomatic nor 'hysterical' in origin. Anxiety and depression, when present (because they are not always so), are likely to be the result rather than the cause of these disabling disorders. The treatment of both disorders is similar, with attention focused on sleep, graduated exercise, medication and diet.

Come back now to Fionnuala. She was told that she had fibromyalgia, and she could see how her sleep, and various other stresses in her life at the time, had contributed to her symptoms. Notwithstanding, she embarked on a ten-day Low Allergy Diet. This improved the quality of her sleep! How interesting, don't you think? It may be that this was the mechanism by which her fibromyalgia improved, for improve it did. Her hands, in particular, were not as stiff or painful; and the awful 'sore all over' feeling was much less than before. Food challenges were then given, one by one, until she had identified all of her safe foods, as well as a few that disrupted her sleep. She now avoids these foods and remains well. Symptoms are apt to return if her sleep is disrupted for any reason.

SECTION 5

Associated Topics

14 The Truth about Candida

Candida has received a great deal of attention in recent years, and has earned a rather dubious reputation in the public mind. It is said to be the cause of an untold number of human ills. All manner of symptoms have been attributed to it, from temper outbursts to impotence. In fact, if you read through the non-medical books on the subject you will find at least fifty different symptoms thus blamed on Candida. The medical community, on the other hand, is not so concerned. It recognises that Candida can cause oral, skin and genital infections, of course, but these respond very rapidly to treatment. It further recognises that patients with compromised immune systems are prone to more serious and widespread Candida infection. Apart from these clearly understood infections, doctors generally consider Candida to be an innocent bystander. Let's take a closer look at this contentious issue.

What is Candida?

Candida is a family of yeast. In fact, it is a rather large family consisting of at least 200 different species, brothers and sisters, so to speak. The most important of these, from a human point of view, is Candida albicans. This yeast inhabits the mouth, gastrointestinal tract, vagina and skin of healthy humans. There is nothing unusual about this, for many micro-organisms inhabit our bodies in this way. The relationship we have with these, our resident microbes, is a symbiotic one: they scratch our back and we scratch theirs. We provide them with a place to live and nutrients to live on; and they, in return, provide us with several important services, including (i) assistance with digestion, (ii) provision of some vitamins, and (iii) some degree of protection from more harmful microbes.

Our resident microbial colonies compete with each other for space and food. This is healthy competition. It ensures that an ecological balance is struck between bedfellows, and in the context of this chapter, it ensures that the Candida yeasts are held in check. The immune system, meanwhile, keeps a watchful, balancing eye on all of this ecological pushing and shoving. In summary, then, we all have Candida. And, in health, it is an innocent bystander. Having thus rescued its reputation, it must be said that Candida can cause several problems: we can be allergic to it, we can be infected by it and we can have too much of it.

Candida allergy

Some people are allergic to Candida, there is no doubt about this. Urticaria, rhinitis and asthma are sometimes triggered by this allergen. The medical literature also contains indisputable descriptions of Candida allergy in the bowel and genitalia. These are less well-known entities, but very real nonetheless.

Candida allergy in the bowel . . .	causes 'mucous colitis', a condition characterised by slimy and sometimes profuse diarrhoea.
Candida allergy in the vagina . . .	causes vaginitis, an inflammation that looks like infection. The symptoms include pain, itch and redness.
Candida allergy on the penis . . .	also causes inflammation. The symptoms are itch, pain and swelling.

Note: In all of these cases, a skin-prick test to Candida will be positive, and the patient will enjoy dramatic symptomatic relief from anti-Candida treatment.

Candida infections

Candida albicans can cause infection under certain circumstances. It changes from a normal inhabitant to an infective agent when the ecological status quo is lost. The most obvious example of this is the vaginal (or oral) thrush that so frequently follows a course of antibiotics. The antibiotic kills the germ it was intended to kill, but it also kills off many innocent bacteria. Candida, on the other hand, being resistant to ordinary antibiotics, grows away happily in their presence. It has no competition from other bacteria, so it just keeps on growing. Before long, it causes symptoms of infection. In this sense, Candida albicans can truly be called an opportunistic agent: it has no ability of its own to invade, and will infect only if given the opportunity to do so. There are three types of opportunistic infection caused by Candida. These are described as superficial, deep and systemic. Deep and systemic (blood-borne) invasions only ever occur in patients who are immuno-compromised, such as patients with AIDS or those seriously ill with some other disease. Superficial infections, by contrast, are very common. As the name suggests, the invasion is limited to superficial layers of the surface being infected. Commonly affected sites include the skin, mouth and vagina; less commonly affected are the linings of the throat, oesophagus, stomach and bowel.

Candida on the skin
Candida infections of the skin may occur at any age, but there are two age groups that are particularly prone. Children under three years of age, for example, easily develop Candida infections in the nappy area, giving them anything from a mild irritation to a rather nasty dermatitis. The second group at risk are adolescents who take antibiotics for recurrent urinary or throat infections, or acne. The principal symptom of Candida infection of the skin is an itchy rash which may, at its worst, become excoriated and sore. Infection most frequently affects the skin folds (where it's warm and moist), such as the armpits, the groin, and the spaces between toes and fingers. The nails, too, may be affected.

Candida in the mouth
Oral infections occur in all age groups, but again, some groups are more at risk than others. Seven per cent of infants, for example, get oral Candida (thrush). They are prone to infection because their immune systems are immature, and they have not had enough time to establish an ecological balance with other friendly microbes. The elderly are also commonly affected, possibly because of the ageing process itself, and in some cases because of ill-fitting dentures. Finally, diabetic patients, whose sugar levels are too high, and patients who inhale steroids for their asthma, are more likely to develop infection. The main symptom of oral thrush is pain, especially when eating salty or spicy foods. Other symptoms include (i) sores at the corners of the mouth, (ii) inflamed mucous membranes inside the mouth, (iii) white creamy plaques on the tongue and on the inner aspect of the lips, cheeks and palate, and (iv) mouth ulcers.

Candida in the vagina

Candida infections in the vagina are extremely common, with 75 per cent of women experiencing at least one bout during their childbearing years. Half of these can expect a second infection at a later date. The universal symptom of vaginal Candida is itch. This may or may not be accompanied by a vaginal discharge which, if present, is said to be white and creamy (a bit like cottage cheese) but which may also assume a watery appearance. Other symptoms include vaginal soreness, painful intercourse, and 'bladder pain' when passing water. The last is frequently mistaken for cystitis (a bladder infection), but this symptom arises from irritation of the bladder neck, rather than from a bladder infection per se. Treatment is usually very successful. Having said that, 5 per cent of adult females are plagued by recurrent or chronic infection. Some of these may be infected with a Candida species other than albicans, such as Candida tropicalis. The latter is rare but becoming more common, and is more resistant to treatment. However, and bearing in mind the fact that Candida is an opportunistic fellow, it is more likely that patients with recurrent infection are struggling with their internal ecological balance. Factors which alter the balance and predispose to vaginal infection include:

- pregnancy
- oral contraceptives, especially those with high doses of oestrogen
- antibiotics, especially the broad-spectrum (blunderbuss) ones
- steroids
- allergy in the vagina, to perfumed toilet paper, for example
- certain diseases, such as diabetes mellitus

Other factors which may be important include:

- tight clothing, especially nylons, which prevent adequate ventilation
- eating lots of sugary foods
- vaginal douches
- swimming in chlorinated pools
- intrauterine contraceptive devices (IUCDs)
- frequency of sexual intercourse
- reinfection from an untreated sexual partner
- reinfection from a reservoir of Candida in the bowel (see below)

Bacterial and other vaginal infections are twice as common as vaginal thrush. The only way to make sure that you are, in fact, dealing with thrush, and not some other infective agent, is by having a vaginal swab test. Also, the symptoms of *allergic* vaginal inflammation are very similar to the symptoms of *infective* inflammation. For this reason allergy is often overlooked, and mistaken for infection. The transient relief which Candida-allergic women enjoy from anti-Candida treatments only adds to the confusion. They feel they must have infection because their symptoms clear up with treatment. The real reason for their relief, however, is the reduction of vaginal Candida as *allergen* rather than as *infective agent.* The clue is the disparity between symptoms and the presence of yeast. Allergic symptoms may be severe in the absence of a significant vaginal discharge, and in the presence of only a small amount of Candida. Patients with recurrent vaginal infections should have a skin-prick test to exclude Candida allergy. They should also read the rest of this chapter!

Candida in the bowel

We have already established that Candida is a normal inhabitant of the bowel, and that its numbers are kept in check by other microbes with whom it must compete. Once again, there are several factors which may upset this balance and predispose to Candida overgrowth. These are:

- being very young or very old
- recurrent pregnancies
- the oral contraceptive pill
- taking antibiotics
- eating a diet of sugary foods
- vitamin deficiency
- having a stomach lacking in acid (hypochlorhydria)
- taking remedies for indigestion or stomach ulcers (antacids)
- taking steroids
- stress

Candida infections in the bowel, as elsewhere, may take on superficial or deep forms, and I stress again that the latter only ever occur in the seriously ill. The symptoms of infection are diarrhoea, flatulence, abdominal pain, rectal bleeding and an itchy bum. No other symptoms occur — except in moribund, and usually hospitalised, patients whose immune defences have collapsed entirely. However, we need to understand that

Candida overgrowth is not synonymous with Candida infection. This is important. They are two different conditions. Infection implies some attempt by the organism to invade tissue; and overgrowth refers simply to a population explosion without invading qualities.

We are particularly interested in this overgrowth phenomenon, because it gives rise to two problems. The first was alluded to above, namely that increased numbers of Candida constitute a rich reservoir for recurrent vaginal infections. Note the sequence of events here. The distance between rectum and vagina is short, and easily breached by the imaginative yeast. To treat the vagina repeatedly whilst ignoring the intestinal reservoir is to fight a losing battle, for no sooner has the vagina been cleared than it becomes infected again through this route. Please also note that hygiene has little or nothing to do with it! Recurrent infections are not a sign of 'dirtiness'; they occur just as frequently in meticulously clean individuals. The one sanitary precaution which females should adopt in this regard is to wipe the bottom from front to back after a bowel movement.

The second major problem of Candida overgrowth is the Gut Fermentation Syndrome. This condition may affect both men and women, and it may occur with or without genital infections. As you shall see, gut fermentation may be caused by any number of different microbes. Candida, although commonly implicated, is just one candidate. There are many other yeasts and bacteria that can drive the fermenting process.

Gut Fermentation Syndrome: intestinal dysbiosis

We have described symbiosis as a relationship of mutual benefit between one organism and another, or between several organisms and a host. In this context, we are talking of the friendly relationship that exists between our bodies and the myriad microbes which live inside us. Indeed, there are an estimated one hundred thousand million microbes in each gram of faeces! In health, these microscopic residents are maintained in a state of balance. If this equilibrium is lost, for whatever reason, one micro-organism will grow at the expense of others. The diplomatic relationship between host and organism is now less harmonious than heretofore. We refer to this as a state of dysbiosis. Furthermore, if the expanding microbe just so happens to be capable of fermentation, it may give rise to symptoms. Several bacteria and yeasts fall into this category. They live by fermenting the sugars in our diet. That is, they set to work on 'eating' the sugars, and they produce alcohol as a by-product.

Some fermentation takes place inside all of us, and there are usually no problems with this. But if the fermenting population becomes unacceptably large, the fermentation process — the feeding frenzy, as it were — also increases dramatically. Now we have a situation where alcohol and other products of fermentation, such as gas and toxins, are released into the bowel. Alcohol and toxins are then absorbed into the bloodstream, from where they cause a lot of misery. In extreme (and very rare) cases, patients have been known to intoxicate themselves by eating carbohydrate foods, i.e. they can get drunk on sugars!

The symptoms of gut fermentation include:

- abdominal pain
- altered stool frequency
- altered stool form
- altered stool passage
- passing mucus from the back passage
- bloating of the abdomen
- itchy bottom
- flatulence
- indigestion

As you can see, these symptoms overlap greatly with those of the Irritable Bowel Syndrome. This has to do with the direct effect of microbial overgrowth and fermentation on bowel function. These are 'local' symptoms. The absorption of alcohol and other toxins into the blood gives rise to 'distant' symptoms, namely

- fatigue
- headache
- muscle pain
- joint pain

Furthermore, some patients attribute their depression, disturbed sleep and impaired concentration to excessive fermentation. Whilst I fully accept that these symptoms are often part of the overall picture, it is difficult to separate them from the reactive effects of feeling ill for so long. However the notion that fermentation causes 'brain symptoms' is not as daft as it may first appear. Acetaldehyde, for example, is a by-product of fermentation and is known to affect a specific (dopamine) receptor in brain cells. In any case, these troublesome symptoms clear up once the fermentation is treated.

You will also appreciate that many of these symptoms may be caused by food intolerance, or indeed any number of other conditions. In days gone by, we had no option but to put patients on a lengthy diet if we suspected they had fermentation; and patients had to wait some considerable time before they knew whether they would benefit from treatment. Our task is now greatly facilitated by the recent development of a blood test.

A blood test for gut fermentation

Microbes produce alcohol when they ferment sugars. Specifically, yeasts produce ethanol,* and bacteria produce butanol and propanol. We can measure these different alcohols in the blood. If the levels are raised we can deduce that excessive fermentation is taking place; and, depending on the type of alcohol produced, we can say whether the fermentation is of yeast or bacterial origin. We cannot specify which yeast or bacterium is responsible for the fermentation, but that's okay — we don't need to know. There is one treatment for yeast fermentation, whatever the yeast; and another for bacterial fermentation, whatever the bacterium. Here are a few examples.

Pauline was a very busy person with a very important job. She was responsible for the day-to-day management of a large company. Over the past five years she had suffered from recurrent vaginal infections. Swab tests confirmed that she was infected with Candida albicans. She had become quite fed up with the vaginal itch and pain. Symptoms persisted in spite of frequent prescriptions from her doctor. Her husband was also treated on a number of occasions 'just in case'. Pauline suddenly became very unwell about six months before she presented to the Allergy Clinic. She was exhausted. She also developed pains in her muscles and joints. Her back, shoulders and arms were affected in this way. At one stage, she was so ill that she slept sixteen hours a day for the best part of three weeks. In addition, she complained of bouts of diarrhoea, abdominal pain, an itchy bottom, and indigestion. She lost a stone in weight.

Throughout this time her vaginal infections continued unabated. In fact, she now had chronic vaginal symptoms. A blood test revealed that Pauline was suffering from the effects of yeast overgrowth in the bowel. She was put on a diet, and she was prescribed anti-fungal medication to take by mouth. One

---

*You may not know it, but you are probably familiar with this alcohol already — it's the intoxicating part of your favourite drink!

month later, and already feeling considerably better in herself, she was given anti-fungal treatment for the vaginal infections. Over the following weeks and months, she expanded her diet, bit by bit. At the time of writing she remains well, and she has had only one bout of vaginal thrush in the past eight months.

Fred, too, was a busy person, and had a very demanding job. Over the previous three or four years he complained of increasing fatigue. He also complained of abdominal symptoms, such as bloating and diarrhoea. He thought that certain foods were making him ill. In particular, he discovered that all forms of sugar affected him. The problem for Fred, however, was his craving for the very foods that 'wiped him out'. He underwent a Low Allergy Diet for ten days and although he felt somewhat better, he still had quite a few symptoms left. It was clear that his problem was not food intolerance. A blood test for fermentation was then arranged. It came back positive. In fact, the alcohol level in his fasting blood was forty times higher than it should have been! He was started on a regime of diet and anti-fungal medication.

Fred simply could not believe the improvement in his health once he controlled his fermentation. It took a little longer in his case because the levels were so high. Pauline and Fred had yeast fermentation. Notice I didn't say they had 'Candida'! Their fermentation may have been caused by Candida, but it may just as easily have been caused by other yeasts in the gut.

Andrea was different. She suffered from recurrent urinary infections, and had taken twenty courses of antibiotic in as many months! During this time she developed many other symptoms, including fatigue, headaches, fitful sleep, impaired memory and concentration, muscle pains and joint pains. Interestingly, she had little by way of abdominal symptoms. However, in view of her inordinate consumption of antibiotics, and the timing of her symptoms, we performed a gut fermentation test. This revealed the presence of bacterial fermentation. Her butanol levels were about ten times higher than they should have been. She was given antibacterial medication (but not an antibiotic!) together with the gut fermentation diet.

Within a month she felt better, and within three months she was back to her old self. When she started to expand her diet again, she reacted to wheat and a few other foods. Thus, Andrea had a combination of gut fermentation and food intolerance. This is quite a common occurrence. And, as you shall see in the next chapter, gut fermentation is also associated with chemical sensitivity.

The treatment of Gut Fermentation Syndrome

The aim of treatment is to restore balance amongst micro-organisms in the gut. To this end, we must reduce the overgrown population to normal numbers. We do not need to eradicate them completely, nor do we want to. We respect that, in the right numbers, they provide us with many benefits. Besides, we couldn't get rid of them all; they're too versatile for that! A simple culling will suffice. To this end we employ four tactics:

1. We restrict our intake of sugars, thus depriving the microbe of its favourite food (and ours!).
2. We use medication to further reduce the microbial population.
3. We replace the fermenting microbe with friendly bacteria.
4. We use nutritional supplements to help our immune systems.

The only difference between the treatment of yeast and bacterial fermentation is in the use of medication. The principles of diet, microbial replacement and nutritional supplement are the same.

The gut fermentation diet

You will find variations on this theme in various books, some of them stricter than others. Mine is fairly relaxed by comparison. The diet applies to both yeast and bacterial fermentation.

Stage 1
For the first month you should eat only the following (preferably fresh) foods:

- Meat   All sorts: lamb, pork, beef, venison, rabbit, etc.
- Poultry   All sorts: chicken, turkey, pheasant, duck, quail, etc.
- Fish   All sorts, including shellfish; but must be fresh, not in batter!
- Vegetables   All sorts, except sweetcorn and peas, which are high in sugar.

    Eat plenty of greens, and garlic (which has known anti-fungal properties). Potato and rice are 'good carbohydrate' foods and should be eaten in moderation — say, two helpings per day. You can also use rice cakes.

- Fruit   Two normal portions of your choice per day.
- Beans and pulses   All sorts, but in moderation: kidney bean, lentils, sunflower seeds, etc.
- Cheese   Edam and Gouda cheese are allowed, as is goat's cheese.
- Live yoghurt   and plenty of it (see below)
- Eggs and butter
- Use olive oil for cooking purposes.
- Drink only bottled (or filtered) spring water, herbal teas, and calcium-fortified soy milk.
- Take medication, nutritional supplements and friendly bacteria as prescribed, and continue on these throughout the entire process (see below).
- Obviously, if you know you are allergic to any of the above, stay away from them!

Stage 2

You should have noticed some improvement in symptoms by the end of the first month. You can now expand your diet. However, some of the improvement may have been due to the fact that you stopped eating food(s) to which you are intolerant. It would be wise then, to introduce these foods one by one, and observe your reaction to them as you do so (see the Low Allergy Diet in chapter 17 for more details on this). Continue to eat all of the stage 1 foods throughout this time, and test each new food as follows:

Day 1:   Cow's milk: drink one glass at each meal for one day.

Days 2, 3 and 4:   Wheat, in the form of:
                    (i)   wholemeal pasta,
                    (ii)   pure shredded wheat,
                    (iii)   wholemeal bread
                 Some form of wheat must be eaten at each meal for the three full days. The bread should ideally be home-made, using wholemeal flour — no white flour added. Use bread soda, and add an egg if you like. You may also use buttermilk, if milk is safe.

Day 5:   Peanuts, in the form of
                    (i)   peanut butter (with no added
                            sugar)
                    (ii)   raw monkey nuts
                    (iii)   salted peanuts
                    Stay away from dry-roasted nuts. Eat
                    some form of peanut at each meal for
                    one day.

Days 6 and 7:   Corn, in the form of:
                    (i)   corn on the cob
                    (ii)   home-made popcorn
                    (iii)   cornflour, to make a sauce
                    Eat some form of corn at each meal
                    for two full days.

Days 8 and 9:   Oats, in the form of
                    (i)   porridge
                    (ii)   oatcakes
                    Eat some form of oat at each meal for
                    two full days.

Days 10 and 11:   Rye, in the form of
                    (i)   Ryvita crispbread
                    (ii)   pure rye bread
                    Eat some form of rye at each meal for
                    two full days.

Stage 3

By now you should be well and truly on the road to recovery. If you are, try out the following over the coming month: all kinds of cheese (including mouldy ones), tea and coffee, all sorts of nuts, and alcohol. Later, you may also venture towards cake, biscuits, chocolate, ice cream, rich sauces, etc.

Please accept two words of warning before we leave the subject of diet. Firstly, if you have not enjoyed obvious and lasting benefit within two months of this regime, *then something is wrong*! The diagnosis should be reconsidered in such cases. Please resist the urge to stay on this, or any other, diet, unless it has been advised by your doctor/dietician. Secondly, watch out for a return of symptoms as you reintroduce sugary foods. These symptoms are likely to creep up on you gradually, as the fermentation builds up. Once again, please get expert help if you find this happening.

I believe that the vast majority of patients with fermentation can end up with a normal, or nearly normal, diet. In other words, gut fermentation is a treatable disorder with a high rate of cure. You would, of course, be well advised to eat a healthy diet for the rest of your days. This will mean some degree of moderation in your consumption of sugars, but it will also allow the occasional splurge!

Drug treatment for gut fermentation

The choice of drug is dictated by the organism we are dealing with. Yeast can be tackled head-on with anti-fungal drugs, whereas we must take a more subtle approach with bacterial overgrowth.

Yeast fermentation

The most effective medicine for the treatment of yeast fermentation is nystatin, a powerful anti-fungal drug. This is taken, ideally, in the form of a powder. All other preparations of nystatin are sugar-laden. Fortunately, nystatin is also a very safe drug, and can be taken in large doses without ill effects. Its safety and efficacy stem from the fact that its absorption into the body is negligible. This serves our purpose well. We want it to stay in the gut.

Some patients complain that nystatin makes them feel ill, and there is no doubt that a minority of these are genuinely intolerant to the drug itself. But most of the symptoms attributed to nystatin actually come from the dying yeast colonies. Yeast cells burst when they die, and their contents spill out into the gut. Some of these substances are toxic to us, and they give rise to flu-like symptoms, such as headache, fatigue, and aches and pains in the muscles. These die-off reactions, as they're called, can be minimised by starting with very small doses of nystatin, with gradual increases until therapeutic (effective) levels are reached. Starting the diet a week before the nystatin will also help, for this will (slightly) reduce yeast populations in itself. Nystatin is a prescription-only medicine, so discuss its use with your doctor. I recommend the following dosage schedule:

Dosing schedule for dry nystatin powder

Start with: 1/8 level teaspoon per day for three days — literally the tip of a level teaspoon

Then double to:	¹/₄ level teaspoon per day for three days
Then double to:	¹/₂ level teaspoon per day for seven days
Then double to:	1 level teaspoon per day. I usually advise patients to stay on this dose for a total of three months, and only rarely have to give larger doses.

Note: The powder does not taste nice! Mix your daily dose into live yoghurt, store it in the fridge, and dip into it several times a day. Die-off reactions may occur when you start nystatin, and at any dose increase thereafter. If you get die-off symptoms, grin and bear them, they will pass. If they're too severe, go back to the previous dose, and try to increase the dose again in another week.

A word about other anti-fungals

Nystatin is the most suitable medication for yeast fermentation, but some patients (a minority) are intolerant to it. They get symptoms even when they observe the dosing precautions just described. These require an alternative anti-fungal. All such treatments are prescription-only medicines. They are absorbed into the bloodstream, and are therefore less effective than nystatin in the treatment of fermentation. They are very effective for the treatment of infection, however. The use of these drugs should be discussed with your doctor. Some individuals and health food shops sell stuff which is supposedly anti-fungal. The truth is, this *limits* the ability of yeast to grow, but it doesn't kill it off. If you have a significant overgrowth you will need a 'killer', not a 'limiter'. Once the overgrowth is controlled, then by all means use these yeast-limiting agents to prevent a recurrence.

Bacterial fermentation

Bacterial overgrowth cannot be tackled head-on with antibiotics; that would only make matters worse! There is one exception to this rule, and that's the young child with severe upper gastro-intestinal overgrowth, who will respond well to antibiotics. For the rest of us, we rely on an old drug, bismuth. This medicine was popular in times past for the treatment of gastritis and ulcers, and is still used today. It is thought to work by lining the stomach with a protective coat. When bismuth lines the stomach and intestine it acts rather like grease on a pole: it's very hard for bacteria to cling onto the bowel wall. They lose their grip, slip off, and get expelled from the body in the faeces. Bismuth should not be taken for longer than three months at a time because it's absorbed into the bloodstream. Two tablets taken half an hour before breakfast and evening meals is the recommended dose. It turns the stool black!

Friendly bacteria to restore the balance

Once we kill off the fermenting organism we must fill the empty space with friendly bacteria. This will ensure that the fermenting organism is held in check. The best way to achieve this is to flood the gut with friendly bacteria, such as those we find in live yoghurt. They go by some wonderful names, such as *bulgaricus*, *lactobacillus* and *bifidus*. Choose a brand that guarantees live bacteria, and eat one good-sized pot of it every day. Some brands boast two or more cultures of bacteria. These are the best, for they provide a variety which can only help the ecological balance of the gut.

You should verify that your chosen yoghurt is truly 'alive' by the following simple test. Place a dessertspoon of milk on top of a newly opened pot of yoghurt, put the top back on, and place it in a warm oven. Come back in five hours and observe that the milk has disappeared. If it hasn't, the 'live' culture is, in fact, dead! Supplements of friendly bacteria are also available. One of the most popular of these is acidophilus. However, beware of the claims — many of the acidophilus are dead by the time they reach your local supplier!

Nutritional supplements to help our immune systems

Yeasts grow more vehemently in the absence of certain vitamins. They also grow more readily in the absence of an effective immune system. The B vitamins are important in this regard, so take a supplement of B complex throughout the diet. Other nutrients may also help, but these should be determined on an individual basis.

Candida Hypersensitivity Syndrome?

I come back now to my opening paragraph, in which I pointed out that all manner of ills have been blamed on Candida. Some practitioners refer to this plethora of symptoms as the Candida

Hypersensitivity Syndrome, or 'candida', for short. Their list is far more extensive than the symptoms I have described above, and there are two sources of confusion here. The first is the commercial interest of unqualified practitioners who forcefully tell clients that their unexplained symptoms are due to 'candida' — and then sell them the wherewithal to treat it! The second is this: the popular treatment for 'candida' involves killing several birds with one stone. Thus, potentially 'allergic' foods (such as wheat and yeast) are avoided; pharmacologically active foods (such as caffeine and alcohol) are avoided; 'tiring' foods (sugars) are avoided; and nutritional supplements are taken in large doses. These measures, *in and of themselves*, would improve the health of many.

Thus, the 'candida regime' could help the food-intolerant, the caffeine-addicted, the hypoglycaemic, the nutritionally deficient and the gut-fermenting. The fact that you improve on a 'candida regime' does not necessarily prove that your symptoms were caused by 'candida', but one can readily understand this source confusion.

You will also notice that all of the symptoms attributed to Candida in this chapter can be verified by clinical and laboratory tests, and by their speedy response to appropriate treatment. I would encourage anyone with persistent symptoms to seek expert help, and, if need be, to think again about the diagnosis of 'candida'. When all is said and done, most patients should end up with a clear understanding of the true nature of their symptoms. This will afford them the best possible chance of obtaining relief.

15   *Chemical Sensitivity*

Man has introduced countless chemicals to his environment since the Industrial Revolution, and continues to add to the tally at a present rate of 1,000 new compounds each year. At least 10,000 of these are in regular use. Each one of us will encounter an estimated 200 man-made chemicals in the course of a normal day, and up to 400 if we live or work in a chemically laden environment. This proliferation of chemical use is now an issue of environmental concern. We have indiscriminately thrown thousands of tons of chemical waste into our water, soil and air.

On a global scale, we have punched a hole in the ozone layer; and at national level, we find many countries in dire straits with uncontrolled pollution. We must not believe for one moment that we can inflict such damage on our environment without incurring some penalty on health. After all, we are an integral part of the environment. We eat the food, drink the water and breathe the air! In so doing, and if I may borrow a phrase, we *internalise* the environment we live in.

We should not think, therefore, in terms of 'the environment' and 'us', but in terms of our external and internal environments as a continuum. We cannot expect to harm one without also harming the other. For example, during the past twenty years industrialised countries have witnessed an alarming rise in allergic diseases, and the finger has been pointed squarely at air pollution as a significant contributing factor to this.

Many pollutants build up in our bodies over time. For instance, PCBs (polychlorinated biphenyls), widely used in the electrical industry, have been detected in the breast milk of nursing mothers. They are thought to contribute to increased rates of infection in the newborn. Likewise, pollutants have been detected in our blood, sweat and urine. There can be little doubt, then, that we are collectively affected by what we throw into our environment.

We also hear of individuals being poisoned in various ways by toxic chemicals: chemical warfare, commercial negligence, occupational and domestic accidents all occur. We have heard of the Gulf War Syndrome, for example, a debilitating condition affecting many veterans of Desert Storm. It is thought to be caused, at least in part, by chemical exposures suffered by soldiers during their tour of duty in the Persian Gulf. Negligent exposures are also well publicised, for example the outbreak of illness amongst seventy people who ate cucumber contaminated with pesticide. In contrast, occupational and domestic accidents receive less attention. The farmer who falls into a sheep-dip, or the gardener who sprays himself with herbicide, are not going to make it into the news! As you shall see, these poisonings may lead to very troublesome illness.

Before we proceed, we should remind ourselves of the other ways in which chemicals are known to affect individual health. In previous chapters we covered chemical allergy as a possible trigger for many conditions, including contact allergic dermatitis, conjunctivitis, rhinitis, asthma, urticaria and anaphylaxis. We also described the non-allergic (irritant) effects of chemicals on these disorders, as well as the chemical intolerance that occurs in some cases of hyperactivity and migraine. In summary, then, we have established that chemicals may give rise to pollutant, toxic, allergic, intolerant and irritant effects. In this chapter, however, I want to address something quite different: I want to talk about canaries!

CASE HISTORY

Rory was a farmer who kept livestock. One day, as he was inspecting his herd, a dreadful accident occurred. A plane, which had strayed off course, flew overhead and doused him with pesticide. He suffered the immediate effects of chemical irritation, and ran back to his house for a shower. By the time he got there, his eyes were red and sore, his nose was burning, and he had developed a hacking painful cough. Some of these symptoms settled after a wash and a change of clothes, but other symptoms soon took their place. His head was pounding, he felt nauseous and his muscles started to twitch. He was admitted to hospital. Although his acute symptoms settled down after a few days, he was left feeling very tired and ill. That was twenty years ago, and Rory has never felt well since. His doctors had no difficulty diagnosing his original illness: he had acute organophosphate poisoning, but they found it more difficult to understand the vague and chronic symptoms which he experienced subsequently. For instance, every time he got a whiff of paint he collapsed to the ground — just fell like a ton of bricks! Sometimes, he would start to shake uncontrollably with muscle spasms. His doctor was called to the scene on more than one occasion to provide emergency treatment. Over the years, Rory started to react in this way to a host of other smells, including perfumes, air fresheners, traffic fumes, and the like. This forced him to adopt a secluded lifestyle, for he could not bear to collapse in front of his perfumed (or aftershaved) friends. Rory has Multiple Chemical Sensitivity — he's a canary!

In times past, miners took canaries down their shafts and kept them in cages close to the coalface. Their reason for doing so was simple, if somewhat cruel. Miners were at risk of poisoning from dangerous gases emanating from the coalface, and they had no way of knowing when the levels were high. Canaries, being very sensitive creatures, react swiftly to changes in their environment. They die in the presence of *relatively low amounts* of toxic gas. A dead canary was a sign to the miners that they too were at risk of poisoning, and that they should leave the mine post-haste. Rory, and others like him, are sensitive to *relatively low amounts* of environmental chemicals, and much lower levels than would be required to cause visible signs of poisoning. These chemically sensitive 'canaries', by their suffering, may be sending a warning signal to the rest of us: 'Clean up your act! Think again about these chemicals! You cannot afford to pollute your environment!'

You may find all of this a little hard to believe. 'After all,' you may say, 'we are talking about polish and perfume, surely they can't make you ill!' Moreover, you may confidently cite the safety declarations of our public health officials. They tell us reassuringly that the chemicals in common use are safe; and that, as long as we take precautions, even the more toxic chemicals can be used without harmful effects. This is, of course, true — in so far as it goes. The same scientists, however, will readily admit that their statements refer only to toxicity, and not to issues of individual sensitivity. They can tell us, for example, that a particular chemical is either poisonous or safe; and that it will, or it won't, cause cancer. When dealing with shades of grey, they can tell us at what dose a safe chemical becomes poisonous. Their confidence is based on the fact that the toxic effect of chemicals can be easily measured. In stark contrast, the subjective claims of chemical sensitivity are much more difficult to assess. They do not lend themselves to the same scrutiny. Similarly, it is difficult to assess the health effects of prolonged exposure to low doses of chemical, or to mixtures of chemicals. The hardy ('miners') amongst us may not be unduly worried about this, but the sensitive ('canaries') most certainly are.

What is Multiple Chemical Sensitivity?

Multiple Chemical Sensitivity is a term used to describe patients who have hypersensitive reactions to many 'otherwise harmless' chemicals. They also react to toxic chemicals at very low doses, far below those expected to cause symptoms in the general population. Many of these patients give a clear history of a single poisonous exposure from which they have never recovered. Others develop the problem after prolonged exposure to lower, non-poisonous levels of chemical. In all cases, patients are left with an extreme sensitivity to ordinary chemical smells, including perfume, aftershave, deodorants, hair gel, make-up, air fresheners, tobacco smoke, exhaust fumes, newspaper print, new fabric, new cars, photocopiers, printers and plastics. The symptoms they complain of are numerous, and include:

- fatigue
- headache (including migraine)
- nausea
- depression and irritability
- mood swings
- anxiety
- impaired memory and concentration
- pains in the muscles and joints
- sleep complaints

In addition, some of these patients have:

- increased heart rate
- high blood pressure
- increased breathing rate (overbreathing)
- food intolerance (see below)

Who gets it?

We have no way of predicting who will become chemically sensitive. It is said to be more common in women, but this difference may be slight. Acute poisoning with toxic chemicals or prolonged exposure to less toxic chemicals are definite risk factors; and indeed, these 'sensitising' events are prerequisites for the disorder. However, not all poisoned patients will develop chemical sensitivity. This suggests that other factors, as yet unknown, increase the risk for some individuals.

Will they grow out of it?

Chemical poisoning, if severe, can lead to permanent health problems in its own right. These are the direct effects of toxicity and they should be distinguished from the symptoms of sensitivity (which may or may not develop after the poisoning). Once they have been sensitised, these patients are likely to retain their sensitivity throughout life. However, with proper care and treatment many patients can enjoy significant relief.

What causes it?

We are not yet sure of the cause of chemical sensitivity. However, we know that chemical poisoning frequently and seriously disrupts nerve pathways in the brain. Furthermore, we recognise that many of the symptoms of the syndrome, including depression and anxiety, are also the *result of brain dysfunction*. This leads us to a very interesting and plausible theory. It goes something like this:

1. There is an initial exposure to chemicals. This may be either sudden or gradual.
2. The chemicals are transported to the brain via the olfactory (smell) nerve and/or the bloodstream.
3. Susceptible people cannot cope with the chemical onslaught.
4. Their brains become saturated, or overloaded with chemicals.
5. Nerve pathways in the brain become sensitised to chemicals. They lose their previous tolerance, and they develop hypersensitive responses to everyday low-level chemical exposures. They react even to chemicals which are unrelated to the initial exposure.
6. Their brains are left in a state of persistent hypersensitivity, and symptoms arise from the disruption that ensues.
7. Many of the symptoms can be understood in terms of the

particular parts of the brain that are affected, including the symptoms of depression and anxiety.

This theory is referred to as neurosensitisation, or time-dependent sensitisation. In most cases, the initial exposure is sudden and poisonous, frequently requiring emergency medical treatment. In other cases, the exposure is much more gradual and subtle.

CASE HISTORY

Mark had worked in the family business all his life. He owned a petrol station and fixed cars, and did so with impunity for many years. However, he developed symptoms in his late thirties, namely headaches, pains in his eyes, sore muscles, general tiredness and 'terrible indigestion'. By now his symptoms were very disabling, and his life had become something of a misery. In fact, he was downright cranky, his sleep was disturbed and unrefreshing, and his concentration was at an all-time low. As he related the story, he gave one interesting clue: his symptoms improved away from work. This could be the simple benefit of rest, of course, but it could equally signify a chemical sensitivity. Mark was advised to go on a 'chemical holiday' (see p. 249). His symptoms improved 'dramatically' during this time. We then organised a phased return to work, being careful to limit his exposure to chemicals. He discovered that he could work in the shop all day, and run the business from there without symptoms. However, his symptoms returned as soon as he started to fill petrol. He had developed chemical sensitivity after many years of low-dose exposure to petrochemical fumes.

Are there any complications?

The lives of chemically sensitive patients are severely disrupted by their need to avoid chemical smells. Moreover, they have a financial burden to bear, in that as many as 70 per cent give up their jobs on account of the illness. They may also run into trouble with their family and friends, who find it difficult to understand this puzzling and controversial disorder. In addition, chemical sensitivity is often complicated by food intolerance.

CASE HISTORY

Consider Abigail, for instance, a 32-year-old scientist. She was working in the research and development department of a multinational firm. One day there was a chemical spillage in her laboratory and she became violently ill. She was admitted to hospital with headache, nausea and muscle pains. That was a year ago, and she has suffered ever since. In particular, she complained of fatigue, depression, anxiety, headaches and muscle spasms. She also developed asthma and rhinitis. Some of her symptoms got worse when she was exposed to chemical smells — even smells we take for granted, such as pot-pourri and perfumed soap.

By the time she presented to the Allergy Clinic, several hospital specialists had reassured her that nothing 'physical' was wrong. By this they meant that they could find no physical explanation for her symptoms. She did not have a brain tumour, her blood was healthy, and she had no obvious signs of disease. She was told that her symptoms were 'functional'. In other words, everything *looked* okay, it just didn't *function* properly.

Antidepressant medication improved her mental state considerably, but she was left with her most troublesome symptoms. Having thus excluded any other explanation for her symptoms, and in some desperation, Abigail went on a ten-day Low Allergy Diet. To her great relief, all of her symptoms improved. She identified the problem foods one by one, and remains well as long as she avoids these. She is also careful to avoid chemical smells, but even these are more easily dealt with now that she is eating the 'right' diet. Abigail had Multiple Chemical Sensitivity, but most of her symptoms were due to the associated food intolerance.

This case introduces us to another important issue, namely the concept of 'total load'. Let me explain. Abigail had a poisonous event from which she developed chemical sensitivity. This in turn led to food intolerance. Thus, she was reacting adversely to many chemicals and — although she didn't know it at the time — several foods. The total load on her system was considerable. When she reduced the load (by avoiding intolerant foods and chemical smells) she was much better able to cope with transient chemical exposures.

What can we do about it?

If you suspect that you are suffering from chemical sensitivity, go on a 'chemical holiday' (see p. 249). The best treatment for chemical sensitivity is avoidance of chemical smells. In fact, therein lies a good rule of thumb: if it smells avoid it! Reduce your 'total load' by the following means:

1. Create a home which is free of chemicals.
    - See box below.
2. Tell your friends!
    - They will need to be aware of the problem if they're to avoid polluting the environment that you have spent so long cleaning up!
3. Check out your other sensitivities!
    - All patients with Multiple Chemical Sensitivity should consider the Low Allergy Diet for food intolerance (see chapter 17).
    - They should also consider the possibility of gut fermentation (see p. 198).
4. Consider a course of desensitisation, it works well for many patients (see chapter 18).

ADVICE FOR THE CHEMICALLY SENSITIVE

1. You will need to recruit the co-operation of all household members to achieve a low-chemical environment.
    - Beware of teenagers who spray themselves in their bedrooms: the fumes will travel!
2. Do not use cosmetics, especially if they are perfumed.
    - Use lemon juice as an astringent.
    - Use olive or baby oil as a cleansing cream.
    - Use peeled and sliced cucumber puréed with one teaspoon of yoghurt as a 'freshener'.
    - Make up a moisturising cream as follows: one tablespoon each of honey, water and olive oil, mixed with one capsule of vitamin E.
    - You might get away with unperfumed hypo-allergenic cosmetics.
    - You might also get away with a baby shampoo.
    - Use unscented stick deodorants.

---

3. Minimise your exposure to soaps, polishes, bleach, etc.
   - Use baking soda or borax as an all-purpose cleaner.
   - Wash windows with vinegar (one tablespoon) in water (a half-pint).
   - Clean the fridge with soda water.
   - Dust with a damp cloth.
   - Polish with beeswax.
4. Do not use air fresheners
   - Use vinegar or baking soda in water; leave it sitting in a saucer in a corner of the room.
5. You will also need to be aware of other chemical sources.
   - Gas fires and cookers, for example, are heavy contaminants. Electric ones are better.
6. Similarly, the central heating boiler may leak tiny amounts of fumes into the atmosphere.
   - Boilers are better housed in a separate building, such as a shed in the back garden.
   - Leave a few feet of fresh air between the flue and your main dwelling.
   - If you have an integral garage, seal the communicating door.
7. Check out your car!
   - Get rid of your old car if it smells of petrol or diesel.
   - But don't buy a new car, they're too smelly; go for something six to twelve months old.
   - Saloons are better than hatchbacks.

Could it be anything else?

Multiple Chemical Sensitivity is said by some to be a psychiatric disorder. They base their assertion on the fact that the condition defies all of the established doctrines of toxicology. They point out that none of these patients has 'tissue pathology' or other visible effects of toxic poisoning. They also remind us that many of these patients are depressed and anxious. However, I trust that these arguments have been adequately addressed in the text above.

There are, of course, occasional patients who wrongly attribute their symptoms to chemical sensitivity. Take the social phobic, for example. She doesn't want to meet people. She's too shy. It is much easier for her to say, 'I cannot go out because I have MCS,' than admit to her real pain. Meeting people makes her feel terribly inadequate. She has very low self-esteem, and doesn't want to be reminded of it. In the same vein, the depressed man may be unhappy or anxious for any number of reasons, but he has learned that men are macho. Men don't cry, and men certainly cannot admit to psychological weakness. It is much easier for him to complain to his doctor about physical symptoms than emotional ones.

The assessment of any patient with suspected Multiple Chemical Sensitivity must, therefore, be compassionate and dispassionate all at once. It is wrong to tell patients that their symptoms are physical in origin when they are in fact psychological. But more of this anon.

16   Allergy and the Psyche

Doctors of old had very little by way of hard science with which to diagnose and treat disease. They were, by our standards, severely disadvantaged. Recent advances in medicine have provided us with some very real benefits in terms of what we can now achieve for many of our patients. However, the enormous strides we have made in research have brought a few problems of their own. One of these is our fondness for reductionism: the practice of dividing something up until it's small enough to study. We start off with noble desires to study a complex being, such as the human body, but it proves impossible to study in all of its complexity. To get around this problem we decide to divide the complex being into several smaller parts. Thus we invent arbitrary divisions between one organ and another, and between one system and another. Then we discover that the organ or system being studied can itself be further divided and reduced. In this way, we delve ever deeper into the mystery of biological life, until we eventually reach the molecular level. At this stage, and in spite of all our genius, we have still managed only to touch the tip of the iceberg.

There are, of course, many good arguments for a reductionist approach to research. It has led to some very exciting discoveries, and it has increased our knowledge base beyond recognition. For this reason, we have now divided the practice of medicine into many different specialities; and further divided specialities into subspecialities. One of the consequences of all this medical science is that we too, as a society, tend to think in reductionist terms. We think of our bodies as being divided into separate organs and systems, and we tend to forget that every single organ and system in the body is inextricably linked with the next.

In this regard, we are not helped by the popularity of dualism — the philosophy of René Descartes (1596–1650). He argued that mind and body were distinct and separate, and that everything in life could be reduced to either one or the other. It is widely accepted that his influence on the development of science was beyond measure — a truth reflected in the persistence with which this question of mind–body has dogged us ever since. Ironically, the reductionism of science has turned dualism on its head. In the very recent past, scientists have discovered interactions *at a molecular level* between mind and body. What goes on in the mind has a very real effect on the body, whether positive or negative. The converse is also true, namely that the body exerts a direct effect on the mind. There is nothing new about this, of course. We have merely rediscovered an ancient truth. Socrates (*c.*469–399 BC), for example, said that 'it is not proper to cure the body without the soul'. This principle was further promoted by Hippocrates, who told his students that 'in order to cure the body, it is necessary to have a knowledge of the whole of things'. These men considered mind and body to be inseparable. In the true sense of the word, they were holistic in their approach to health and disease. We have come full circle, I hope.

Let us now take a closer look at the molecular interactions between mind and body. Our attention will be focused on the relationship that exists between brain and immune systems. You will soon discover that these systems are inseparable from each other, and from other systems in the body. They are all indivisibly one. In the light of this, the constant squabbling over the psychological (mind) or physical (body) nature of symptoms may be seen as nothing more than a barren remnant of dualism.

Interactions between mind and body

The following diagram shows, rather simplistically, the interaction that occurs between the central nervous system (brain), endocrine system (hormones) and immune system. The shaded area in the middle represents the inseparable nature of these systems.

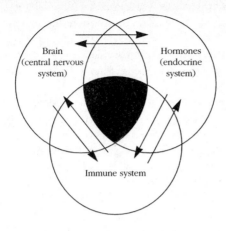

Throughout the body, messages are transmitted from one cell to another by a system of chemical messengers and receptors. Messengers of various kinds are released into the gap between two adjacent cells, or travel in the bloodstream to more distant sites in the body. Receptors of various kinds are found on the surface of cell walls. They are specific, and will respond only to the messenger they were designed to recognise. One cell can talk to another if it stimulates it with the right chemical messenger. We now know that the brain interacts with the immune system in this way. One can talk to the other at a molecular level! In the same way, chemical pathways exist for immune–endocrine and brain–endocrine communication. Thus, one can easily see how an unhealthy brain, for instance, can send 'negative' messages to the immune system, and vice versa.

The effects of mind over body

Doctors of antiquity recognised a link between the psychological state of their patients and the diseases they suffered. For example, in the second century AD, Galen suggested that depressed women were more prone to cancer than women of happier disposition. Throughout medical history, and up to the present day, Galen's preliminary observations have gained support: both men and women may be at risk of cancer after prolonged periods of depression. There also appears to be a link between psychological states and other conditions, such as autoimmune disease and recurrent infection. You will notice that all of these physical manifestations of disease have one common bond: they are failures of immunity. As we discussed in chapter 2, cancer is a failure of immune surveillance, autoimmune disease is a failure of immune judgment, and recurrent infection is a failure of immune response. It is understandable then that some patients going through stressful life events reflect this stress in their immune systems.

Before we proceed to the specific effects of stress on the immune system, we should clarify what it is we mean by stress. A stressful life event is one which requires a person to change. Change demands adjustment, and adjustment is stressful. Our ability to handle adjustment will determine, in large part, how we cope with the stressful event. On the scale of things, the most challenging of all life events is the death of a spouse, with divorce and separation coming second and third respectively. Other stressful events, in order of importance, include enforced detention (hostages, prisoners of war or state, etc.), the death of a (non-spouse) family member, personal injury or illness, marriage, losing your job, and retirement. There are, of course, many other stressors in life, including financial strain, having children, changing jobs and moving house. Finally, there are some stresses which may not be immediately obvious, such as going on holidays, family get-togethers and even Christmas!

You will notice that the most demanding stresses are those which by their very nature are prolonged and uncontrollable. Bereavement is the prime example of this. The grief process takes time, even years, to complete. It cannot be hurried, and there is absolutely nothing that the bereaved can do to bring back their loved one. In this sense they have no control over their grief. This is in stark contrast to some other forms of stress, such as the stress of preparing for an exam, for instance. This is finite stress. There is a date fixed for the exam and come what may, the stress will be over on that day. Furthermore, this stress is controllable. There is a lot the student can do to lessen anxiety. There is a syllabus to study, lectures to attend, tutors to talk to and past papers to consult, all of which helps the student prepare for the exam. Lifestyle can also be adapted to promote chances of success. A schedule which devotes adequate time to study, sleep, exercise and a healthy diet can give the student a feeling of some control in their situation. Finally, there is a reward at the end, not a lifetime of adjustment.

Yet even this transient and controllable stress exerts a direct adverse effect on the immune system: students have lowered immunity leading up to their exams! This effect has been measured in their blood. They have higher levels of antibody to the glandular fever and the cold sore (herpes) viruses.

Let's take a look at the immune effects of some other stressful situations. We know, for example, that . . .

- immunity is low after bereavement, and normalises within twelve months. This fits with the observation that persons going through bereavement are more prone to infection, particularly during the first year of grief.
- separation and divorce also lead to lowered immunity
- those who care for ill relatives are themselves at risk of stress-related illness. For example, children looking after parents with Alzheimer's disease are at risk of depression and infection.

As you can see, the net effect of stress on the immune system is *suppression*, i.e. lowered immunity. Furthermore, stress has a cumulative effect. We have no safety valve, so to speak, by which it can escape. Thus, if we experience several stressful events simultaneously, or in quick succession, we are more likely to suffer greater degrees of immuno-suppression, and more likely to succumb to illness. This is true of all of us, not just the 'weak' or vulnerable. Indeed, vulnerability to stress and depression, in itself, is just another manifestation of mind–body–mind interactions. For instance, children who are bereaved before the age of ten years are at greater risk of depression in later life. So too are those who have had other traumatic life events in childhood. Similarly, adults who have had an episode of major depression are at greater risk of subsequent depression even though the original stressor (the reason for their depression) has passed.

Their vulnerability arises directly from the biological effects of the first episode of depression or trauma. Negative messages are etched into the brain at a molecular level, they are encoded into the very biochemical processes of brain cells. Younger patients are particularly vulnerable because their brains are still developing at the time of the stressful event. This is another example of sensitisation. These unfortunate people are sensitised to depression *by depression*. Once sensitised, they are at risk of depression when they are going through even minor stress. The most severely affected will experience depression spontaneously, in the absence of any stress whatever. It may be difficult for these people to maintain an optimistic mental outlook on life. In contrast, those who have been fortunate enough to emerge relatively unscathed from childhood into adult life would appear to be better placed. They can better cope with life's difficulties if and when they arise. They also enjoy an immune benefit, for we know that . . .

- people who cope well with stress have better immunity than people who find it harder to cope, and
- people who have positive attitudes to stressful life events have better immunity than those with negative attitudes

'Well, that's all very interesting,' you may say, 'but what has this got to do with allergy?' It stands to reason that if psychological stress can affect all of these functions of immunity, it should also affect allergy. Remember, allergy (hypersensitivity types 1 to 4) is also a function of the immune system: in this case, an inappropriate response to an 'otherwise harmless' substance. The link between mind and allergy was first demonstrated, in 1886, by Sir James Mackenzie. He was chatting with a patient who knew she was allergic to roses, and when he produced an artificial rose, which she thought was real, she started to sneeze! Don't go jumping to conclusions now, she really was allergic to roses, but *on this occasion* her response was a psychological one. The symptoms were very real, *they were the symptoms of allergy*, but they were psychologically driven. This was a Pavlovian response.

Remember Pavlov? He rang a bell every time he fed his dogs, and they quickly learned to associate the sound of a bell with the arrival of food — so much so that they started to salivate every time they heard the bell, even in the absence of food. They had been conditioned to respond in this way. A similar phenomenon can be seen in allergy. Take a guinea pig, for example, and expose him to an allergen. The allergen will cause a release of histamine into his blood. Every time you expose him to the allergen, let him also get a smell of something. In no time at all, the guinea pig will release histamine every time he gets the smell, *even in the absence of allergen!*

Come back now to Sir James and his patient. Her brain sent a signal to her nose and it responded as if it were in the presence of allergen. This was a clear manifestation of psychosomatic conditioning. The symptom is experienced in the body (*soma*), but it originates in the mind (*psycho*). We have already discussed one mechanism by which such a reaction may occur when we described the neurogenic inflammation of non-allergic non-infective rhinitis: nerves can mediate inflammation. But now we also know that histamine can be released by a brain signal! Other examples of mind-over-'allergy' include the well-known stressful exacerbations of asthma, urticaria, eczema and migraine, to name but a few. We cannot, with our current knowledge, be sure of the molecular mechanisms by which these exacerbations occur, but we can take note of the clinical observation that they do. This is not to say that allergies are imaginary — they're not! But as you can see from the following list, many allergic conditions have been traditionally thought of as having a psychosomatic component.

Conditions known to have a psychosomatic basis include:

Acne	Irritable Bowel Syndrome
Allergies in general	Itchy bottom
Angina	Peptic ulcers
Angioedema	Skin diseases
Asthma	Tuberculosis
Headaches (including	Urticaria
migraine)	Many others, far too numerous to list
High blood pressure	
Immune disease	
(e.g. rheumatoid arthritis)	

The fact that so many allergic/intolerant syndromes are influenced by the psyche merely reflects the extent to which brain–immune interactions occur. I have deliberately included tuberculosis in this abbreviated list to emphasise a very important point: psychosomatic does not mean 'all in the mind', it means the psyche plays a *role* in the condition. In some cases the psychological influence is important in the initial stages of contracting the disease; at other times it has an effect on the course which a disease will take, once established. As far as tuberculosis is concerned, it takes only one tubercle to give infection, but only one in ten people who are exposed to the tubercle will develop the infection. The others fight it off. This indicates that several factors are important in determining whether a patient succumbs or not. One of these could be nutritional status, for example, but another is the psychological state of the patient. Indeed, it is widely acknowledged that psychological factors play a role in virtually every single condition which patients present to their doctors. As you can see, allergy is no exception to this. An understanding of psyche–soma interactions will only help in the overall management of allergic conditions.

Putting it all down to stress: a note of caution

As discussed in chapter 12.III many patients testify that they have been dismissed as being 'just stressed out' or 'depressed', when they know they are not, and are subsequently proven right. It is dangerous to dismiss a symptom simply because it defies understanding. To do so is to contribute to the most common mistake in medicine, namely the assumption of psychological illness when physical signs cannot (yet) be found.

Symptoms as symbols

Before we leave the question of mind over body, I would like to offer a few provocative thoughts. It concerns the physical expression of disease. If mind and body are inextricably linked, as I believe they are, do physical symptoms merely reflect the psychological ones? Or, to put it another way, are physical symptoms simply a manifestation of the psychological state? Nausea, for example, is a physical manifestation of anxiety with which we are all familiar. It is such a common experience that we have given it a place in our vernacular. 'I'm worried sick,' we say, when we have butterflies in our stomach and cannot face our food. But what about the symbolism of other, less obvious symptoms? I don't want to push this too far (for to do so would be to fall back into the reductionist trap) but I have been struck by several cases which make me wonder.

One of these was a woman who presented to me when I was still a very young doctor in training. She complained bitterly of back pain. I did the usual bits and pieces but failed to bring any relief to the situation. She returned a few days later with her husband, and complained again about back pain. I suggested a new treatment. She then started to argue with her husband, and he became quite abusive. She matched him insult for insult, and then suddenly turned to me and shouted, 'You see, doctor, he just won't get off my back!' I had the clear impression that all treatments directed against her back would fail, and that we should now look at the relationship which she found so back-breaking!

Another case that comes to mind is in some ways similar, and in others quite different. This was a woman in her forties who presented with asthma and rhinitis; it was her first encounter with these symptoms. She couldn't breathe through her nose, and she couldn't take a proper breath into her chest. She was demure, ladylike, quietly spoken, and uptight. We looked for allergic aspects of her condition, but there were none. We then got chatting about life in general. It transpired that her parents were in crisis, with failing health and a wayward son. They had put this woman under a lot of pressure to return to the family home 'just for a while, until things settle down'. That was eight months ago, and she was still there. She described how she was being sucked into the old family psychodynamics, the unhealthy relationships that had so spoiled her childhood. 'How do you feel about that?' I asked. 'I feel I can't breathe,' she replied.

I also remember an elderly patient who had spent some time under a very cruel regime as a prisoner of war. He developed chronic idiopathic urticaria shortly after his release, and that was many years ago now. He was still troubled, he told me, 'by a constant undermining and frustrating itch'. He could find no rest with it. 'It annoys me in my sleep, and during my every waking moment,' he said. When I enquired about the possibility that it was related to the stress of his wartime experience, he shot me down angrily. He had never spoken about that to anybody, and he wasn't about to start now! His face tightened with resolve, and he glared at me, fully expecting a change of subject. It was clear that I had niggled him, and although I fully respected his right to silence, I suspected that this great burden of unspeakable suffering was 'constantly' present with him, and that it 'undermined and frustrated' him greatly. It would also unsettle his sleep and intrude into his every waking moment.

The effects of body over mind

I am constantly amazed at the efficiency of antidepressants in the treatment of depression. If nothing else, the elevation of mood which results from their judicious use clearly shows the 'physical' nature of depression. A physical agent, a drug, can bring about a beneficial effect on the psyche. The depression itself is often the result of stressful life events, and the adverse circumstances may still exist, but that does not prevent a response to physical treatment. I am not hereby advocating the indiscriminate use of antidepressants for every 'touch of the blues', and I personally favour the use of counselling to achieve better coping strategies in the face of stress, but that's not the point. The point is that 'physical' and 'psychological' are again seen to be intertwined. There are many other examples of this. In fact, over 200 prescription drugs — from the oral contraceptive pill to blood pressure tablets — are capable of altering the mood in some way. Similarly, alcohol, a social drug, has immediate and well-known effects on the psychological state; and illicit drugs such as marijuana and heroin, apart from their mood-altering effects, are known to provoke psychosis in susceptible people.

Psychological symptoms may also arise from physical disease. I am not talking here about a patient's psychological reaction to physical disease, but about the fact that the molecular process of disease can cause psychological symptoms. There are many examples of this:

- Depression may precede an emerging Parkinson's disease or cancer by many months, long before the patient knows they are ill.
- Depression may be caused by an underactive thyroid gland.
- Anxiety may be caused by an overactive thyroid gland.
- Anxiety may be the first symptom of anaphylaxis etc.

I could go on and on! Delusions, hallucinations and even personality disorders can all be induced by physical disease. We call them Organic Brain Syndromes, which is just another way of saying body–mind syndromes. These are 'psychological' symptoms driven by 'physical' mechanisms. Specifically, they are the result of immune–brain and endocrine–brain interactions. Remember, psychosomatic symptoms originate in the psyche and are felt in the soma. These symptoms, in contrast, originate in the soma and are felt in the psyche, they are somatopsychic. In the light of this, we can no longer say that depression is just 'all in the mind'!

Throughout this book you will have come across many cases of somatopsychic 'allergy'. Hyperactive children and depressed or fatigued adults who improve on a Low Allergy Diet fall into this category. The depression and anxiety that so often complicate chemical sensitivity and gut fermentation may be considered in the same vein. Once again, we have to admit that we cannot understand the precise molecular mechanisms by which these interactions occur, but we respect the clinical observation that they do. Indeed, there may be other somatopsychic effects still to consider. Why, for instance, do a minority of autistic children improve on a Low Allergy Diet? The possibilities are interesting to say the least. One of them relates to gluten. This food molecule is, in fact, a very complicated piece of work. When eaten by healthy individuals, it is broken down into smaller parts called peptides, and thence to even smaller parts, called amino acids. Gluten peptides behave like opioid peptides, substances with opium-like activity! If an autistic child was lacking the enzyme to break down these opioid peptides, they could build up in the blood and exert a direct effect on brain function. There *is* a group of autistics who have high levels of gluten peptides in their urine and low levels of enzyme in their blood.

We may eventually unravel the mechanisms of somatopsychic fatigue or depression by discovering similar defects in this or other enzyme pathways. Similarly, we may discover why it is that some patients become anxious and overbreathe when they eat something they are intolerant to. However, and as interesting as it is, the wise and impartial reader will want to know what role the placebo effect plays in all of this. This is a reasonable request, and it should be treated with respect.

The placebo effect

A young doctor once had a patient who lay helpless in bed, day after day, with strange symptoms. Every possible investigation was performed in search of an underlying cause but none was found. One morning, the doctor approached his patient and told her that he had finally figured out a cure. He injected her with sterile water. Later that day, the patient told the ward round that she hadn't felt so well in weeks, and that the injection, whatever was in it, had a great effect. This was a placebo response. The patient improved because the doctor told her she would, and she believed him. The doctor now thought that he had discovered the true nature of her symptoms, namely that they were 'all in her head'. Apart from the highly questionable ethics of such a deception, he couldn't have been further from the truth. He didn't understand the manifold facets of the placebo effect. He knew, of course, that any improvement felt by the patient would have to be a placebo effect, for there is nothing pharmacologically active about sterile water. But he was wrong to conclude that the symptoms were imaginary. He failed to appreciate the full extent of the power which mind can have over body, and that very real physical symptoms (as well as imaginary ones) can also be improved by placebo.

He didn't know, for example, that 30 per cent of post-operative patients will experience pain relief when given a placebo, and no one would suggest for a moment that these patients were not in pain! Their pain was as real as it gets. Their response to an inactive placebo (coloured sugar tablets) simply demonstrates the power of suggestion. If I take something which I believe will kill my pain, it has a good chance of killing my pain — not because it is a painkiller, but because I *believe* it is a painkiller, and my belief has a direct and measurable biological effect in my brain. Once again, the thought processes become encoded into the biochemical processes of the brain. In this placebo mental state, I produce my own opium-like substances. They're called endorphins (*endo*, from within, and *orphins*, referring to morphine-like). If I am given a drug which blocks my endorphin receptors, the placebo effect will fail. So, the placebo effect is just another manifestation of the indivisibility of mind and body. Another famous example of the placebo effect is the amazingly low level of painkillers required by soldiers injured in battle. They are happy to be alive and homeward bound. Their overwhelming sense of relief lifts them far above their pain.

Placebos are used in research to tease out the psychological benefits of treatment from the active ingredients of a drug being tested. Patients with a particular condition are randomly divided into two groups. One receives the active drug; the other receives a placebo, usually a sugar tablet. A double-blind trial is one in which neither doctor nor patient knows active from placebo; a single-blind trial is one in which only the doctor knows what the patient has received. These trials are greatly promoted as the only method of validating whether a particular treatment is of any real use. If it is more effective than the placebo, it is effective; if it is no better than the placebo, it is not. Placebos are also used to compile an accurate profile of drug side effects. Patients taking placebo during drug trials do complain of side effects! It can be assumed, then, that patients taking the active drug will also experience side effects, not only because of the drug itself, but because of their anxiety about the drug.

The question must now be asked about the placebo effect in the allergic and related disorders. We know, from Sir James above, that it can and does occur. In fact, it can occur in any branch of medicine and with virtually any condition. The sceptic will ask about your improvement on the Low Allergy Diet. Does it really mean that you have food intolerance? Similarly, your improvement on chemical avoidance or on gut fermentation regimes does not necessarily prove that these were the cause of your symptoms. The only real 'proof', if you need one, is that placebo effects are not lasting. They fizzle out! It may take days, weeks or even a few months, but fizzle out they will. That's why the cases in this or any other literature will be published only when they have been tested by the passage of time. The very fact that this book is so full of such cases is a testimony to the reality of the disorders described herein, and the efficacy of appropriate treatment. As doctors, we would like to subject our theories to the double-blind trials mentioned above; but you will appreciate that the conditions are too complex, and the responses to treatment too individual, for such reductionism. We are content therefore to continue working with clinical observation and experience.

SECTION 6

Allergy Tests and Treatment

17   *Making Sense of Allergy Tests*

Thomas Willis was the personal physician of Charles II in the mid-seventeenth century. He was one of those brave men who had to practise medicine without the help of laboratory tests, and with nothing to rely on but his clinical skills. He and his colleagues became masters in the arts of history taking, observation and physical examination — skills which they have handed down to us. One day he made a discovery: the urine of diabetic patients tasted 'sweet like honey'! This was one of the first clinical tests ever described, and doctors were advised to use it regularly to help them formulate a diagnosis. Nowadays, thankfully, we don't have to taste urine to diagnose diabetes; we use a nice clean chemical test to detect the presence of sugar in urine and blood. We also have access to many other laboratory tests. These help us to confirm or refute our clinical diagnoses.

For a diagnostic test to be useful it must be reasonably sensitive and specific. The ideal test would be 100 per cent sensitive and 100 per cent specific, but the ideal hardly ever exists in medicine. We are content therefore, in checking for disease, to make use of any test which will be (i) positive in almost all cases where the disease is present, and (ii) negative in almost all other cases. In other words, we are looking for a test which will give very few false positives or negatives. In clinical practice, we combine history taking, observation, physical (and mental state) examination, and the results of *reliable* tests to make a diagnosis. To repeat the words of my wise old colleague, 'Allergy tests should not be relied upon to tell us what we didn't know, they should be used only to confirm our clinical suspicions.'

When it comes to allergy, there are several diagnostic tests to help us. These are:

1. blood tests for IgE allergies

2. skin-prick and intradermal tests for type 1 allergies
3. patch tests for contact allergies
4. dietary tests for food intolerance
5. chemical 'holidays' for chemical sensitivity
6. a blood test for gut fermentation

1. Blood tests

The only reliable blood tests for allergy are those which measure IgE. But even here one must exercise care in making a final judgment. We have seen the need for this time and again throughout this book. The most widely used blood test is called the RAST. Don't ask what the letters stand for, but rest assured, it's good hard science! The test can measure the amount of IgE in your blood, and can determine which allergens your IgE is recognising. As reliable as it is, a negative RAST does not exclude allergy.

2. Skin-prick tests

The first skin-prick test, like so many discoveries in medicine, was accidental. A physician watched his cat cross the lawn and come to his side. The cat scratched him and he quickly developed a hive at the site of the scratch. He had the powers of observation to realise that it was the grass on the cat's claw, and not the cat itself, which had caused the reaction, for a clean scratch would produce no hive.

Skin-prick tests are very reliable. The procedure is relatively simple and can be done in the medical office, taking no more than twenty minutes to complete. Many different allergens can be tested at the same time. A drop of each allergen is placed on the skin of the upturned forearm, and the underlying skin is pricked, through the drop, with a tiny (1 mm) lancet. This puts a minute amount of allergen in contact with the mast cells in the skin. If the mast cells are lined with IgE to that particular allergen, they will burst. This gives rise to a hive (a spot of urticaria). As you know, antihistamines block the urticaria response, so the patient must be free of antihistamine medication for the test to be reliable. In general, we can say that 'the larger the reaction, the more significant the allergy'. Allergy Clinics throughout the world will differ considerably in terms of what they screen for. This merely reflects the difference in prevailing allergens between one country and the next. My preference is to test for:

Grass pollens
Weed pollens
Tree pollens
Silver birch pollen
House dust mites
Feathers
Sheep's wool
Cladosporium, alternaria
and other moulds

Trichophyton (the fungus of athlete's foot)
Cat allergen
Dog dander
Horse hair
Cattle hair
Any other allergen suggested by the history

You will notice that all of these allergens are airborne, with the exception of Candida. Even the athlete's foot allergen may become airborne, especially when removing socks!

We can also use the skin-prick test for type 1 allergies to food. However, we exercise great care when dealing with patients who have had serious or potentially serious allergic reactions. In these cases, we test only for one food or a few foods at a time. It is also wise to dilute such allergens, sometimes to a dilution of 1 in 15,000. This will reduce the chances of provoking a serious allergic reaction during the test itself. If the 1 in 15,000 test is negative we increase the dose, in fivefold steps, until we get a positive skin reaction. If the full dose of allergen is still negative, we proceed cautiously to intradermal tests.

Intradermal skin tests

An intradermal test involves the injection of allergen between two layers of skin. This delivers a larger dose of allergen to the mast cells, giving them every possible opportunity to react. If there is still no reaction, we proceed to a dietary challenge. We smear a tiny amount of allergen onto the patient's lip, and we wait. Then, if there is no reaction, we make the patient eat a small amount of allergen, and we wait. We increase the dose of allergen over time until the patient has eaten a normal portion of the suspect food, or until such time as the patient reacts. Needless to say, this procedure is time-consuming and potentially dangerous. It should be done only under medical supervision, and with the right emergency treatment available.

3. Patch tests for contact allergy

Patch-testing involves the careful placement of suspected allergens on the skin of the patient's back (or outer arm). In most cases, the patch is left in place for forty-eight hours. During this time, the patient takes special care not to wet the patch by perspiration or washing. Thus, no showers, baths or swimming. No hard work either! The patch is then peeled off and the first result is obtained. A positive reaction is characterised by redness, swelling and blistering of the skin under the patch. The allergist must distinguish this from an irritant reaction. The patient returns to the clinic two days later for the second (ninety-six-hour) reading. This visit is to pick up 'late' reactions. Unless there is good reason to suspect an unusual (occupational) allergen, we use a screening panel which contains the most common culprits. This panel is known as the Standard European Battery for patch tests. Although you may not recognise most of the named allergens in the following list, you will recognise the materials they are found in (and with which you have the most contact).

(i) *Potassium dichromate.* Possible contact in practically all trades and household products: blue and black inks and dyes, tanned leather, impregnation and corrosive for textiles and furs, wood, cement, paint industry, chromium salts (electroplating), welding fumes, laboratory and photographic chemicals.

(ii) *Neomycin sulphate.* Aminoglycoside antibiotic. Found in many medicaments for external use: creams, powders, ear and eye drops, etc. May cross-react with other aminoglycosides (kanamycin, framycetin, gentamicin, and streptomycin).

(iii) *Thiuram mix.* Vulcanisation accelerator in rubber processing industry for rubber products of all kinds: boots, shoes, gloves, belts, masks, bathing caps, condoms, pessaries, balloons, tubes, adhesive tape, gummed tapes, stethoscopes, catheters, sponges, elastic bandages, antiseptic sprays, tyres, gaskets, saddles and rubber handles. Also occurs as a preservative in insecticides, animal repellents, technical oils, scabies treatments, fungal treatments, alcohol deterrent, antidote against nickel poisoning.

(iv) *Paraphenylenediamine.* Hair dye, leather dye, fur dye, some photocopiers, printing colours.

(v) *Nickel (and cobalt).* Costume jewellery, zip fasteners, eyeglass frames, metal eyelets in shoes, silver, white gold, knives, forks, other kitchen utensils, hairpins and curlers, metal lipstick holders, coins, door handles, thimbles and needles, scissors, writing implements, etc. May also occur in bleaching agents, hair dyes and cement.

(vi)   *Benzocaine.* Commonly used local anaesthetic. May be found in cold cures, cough medicine, painkillers, astringents, sunscreen agents, disinfectants, wart remedies, appetite suppressants, athlete's foot remedies.

(vii) *Formaldehyde.* Production of plastics and synthetic resins used in chipboards, surface treatments and insulation foam. Disinfectants in hospitals, laboratories and sterilisation of instruments; fixative and preserving solutions for histology and anatomy preparations. Disinfectant and preservative in cosmetics of all kinds, including shampoo, bathing foam, deodorants, mouthwash, nail varnish, soap, creams, etc. Also in pharmaceutical ointments, powders, lozenges, gargles, antiperspirants, etc. In industry: glues, oils, drilling fluids; textile, fur, and leather finishes and conditioners; photographic chemicals.

(viii) *Colophony.* Consists of different resin acids. Found in paper, cardboard, plasters, adhesive tapes and glues, polishes and waxes, cosmetics (nail varnish, depilatories, lipstick, make-up, etc.), external medicaments, and dental compounds. Also found in synthetic rubber products, floor coverings, varnishes, paints, sealing compounds, siccatives, solder, brewery pitch.

(ix)   *Quinolone mix.* Ointments and pastes against fungal skin infections, topical anti-inflammatory preparations, wound healing preparations.

(x)   *Balsam of Peru.* In numerous topical medicaments for external use; as fragrance in cosmetics, tobacco, dental materials, oil colours.

(xi)   *Isopropyl-phenyl-paraphenylenediamine.* In black rubber (tyres), rubber gloves, bands, boots and masks.

(xii) *Wool alcohols.* Topical ointments, cosmetics, soaps, shampoo, lipstick, printing ink, furniture polish, technical liquids, metal sealant, impregnation of textile and leather, ski wax, wire insulators.

(xiii) *Mercapto mix.* Rubber products of all kinds: tyres, hard rubber, textile gum, rubber components of shoes and boots, etc.

(xiv) *Epoxy resin.* Used in industry: electrical, plastics, orthopaedic and dental appliances, pacemakers and spectacles, casting moulds, glues, paints (especially underseal, enamels, metal paint, cement and stones), glass fibre strengthened plastics, building materials.

(xv) *Parabens.* Mostly used as preservatives in pharmaceuticals and cosmetics. Both ingested and topical medicaments may contain parabens. Creams, lotions, make-up, lipstick, soaps, sunscreen agents, depilatories, aftershaves. Also occurs in food: marinated, cooked and fried fish products, mayonnaise, spiced sauces, salad dressings, fish pastes, marzipan. May also occur in technical oils, glues, shoe polishes.

(xvi) *p-BPF resin.* As a glue in shoes, leathers, watch straps, belts, rubber articles, stonework sealing, cars, false fingernails, prostheses and glass wool.

(xvii) *Fragrance mix.* Cosmetics (aftershave, pomades, mouthwashes, perfumes, lipstick, sprays, make-up, etc.); medicaments, industrial fluids and cleansing agents. Also occurs in food: ice cream, chewing gum, bread, cakes, sweets, toffee, chocolates.

(xviii) *Ethylenediamine dihydrochloride.* A stabiliser in medication (e.g. theophyllines). Also in: chemical industry, anti-corrosive agent in paint, colour developer, hardening agent in resin, rubber, fungicides and insecticides, synthetic waxes.

(xix) *Quaternium.* Ointments, creams and lotions; cosmetics of all kinds, colourings and polishes.

(xx) *Isothiazolins.* Cosmetics, softeners, glues, watercolours, polish, and wood treatments

(xxi) *Mercaptobenzothiazole.* Rubber products, technical cuttings oils, wires, fungicides, veterinary medical preparations.

(xxii) *Primin.* The allergen of *Primula obconica.* Occurs in primulas and primroses, and cross-reacts with some orchids, jacaranda, teak, and natural sponges.

4. The Low Allergy Diet for Food Intolerance

Imagine the following predicament. You are wandering forlorn in a labyrinth of constant illness. At this point in the maze you come face to face with a door. It's locked, but you can see the light of day through a peephole. You have to figure out a way to unlock the door, so you take a closer look. You can see five handles on your side, but you cannot see which one is keeping the door locked. You decide to try them one by one. You pull down on the first handle and push. Resistance. You let the first one go, believing it to be unimportant, and you pull down on the second. Resistance again. You try all of the handles in this way and, alas, the door remains firmly closed. Then you have a brainwave — perhaps two or more handles are keeping the door locked! So, you take off your scarf and you tie all the handles together. You pull down, opening all five simultaneously, and you're free!

There is only one way to get free from the labyrinth of food intolerance: stop eating all of your regular foods at the same time. There is no point in trying to figure out the 'handles' one by one, you are likely to get confused. Think about it. You exclude one food from your diet, symptoms persist, you put that food back (believing it to be unimportant) and you exclude another, but symptoms persist, and so on. You never manage to unlock the door that keeps you ill. A total fast would in some ways be the ideal approach, but that brings a few problems of its own. Fasting deprives the immune system of its raw material, so to speak, and it cannot keep up an inflammatory response on an empty stomach. Symptoms may therefore improve, but they will recur as soon as food is eaten again, whatever the food. In practice, therefore, we allow ten or twelve foods that (i) are known to be of low allergy potential, and (ii) are not eaten regularly by the patient.

Dietary investigation for food intolerance, stage 1

A word of caution. Young boys with moderate or severe eczema should not do this diet without the close supervision of a medical doctor with an interest. They are at risk of serious reactions during the reintroduction of milk, even if they have never experienced such a reaction before. Migraineurs who have lost the power of an arm or a leg or who have experienced severe visual disturbance during a migraine attack should also be closely supervised. They could get the worst migraine of their lives!

Finally, it is imperative to ensure that all patients end up with a diet that is both nutritionally and socially acceptable. Nobody should be forced to adhere to a restricted diet if the benefit is not obvious to all. If dietary restriction is necessary, get expert dietetic advice to ensure an adequate intake of calories, calcium,

and so on. Bear in mind that once you have identified your culprit foods, there is an effective treatment available to increase
your tolerance to them (see chapter 18).

A typical Low Allergy Diet starts off with the following
(preferably fresh) foods: lamb, salmon, cod, trout, plaice, broc-
coli, parsnip, sweet potato (sometimes called 'yams'), turnip,
courgette, kiwi, pears. Use olive oil for cooking. Drink only bottled spring water — natural or carbonated.

During stage 1, remember:

- It may be preferable to conduct the diet under medical supervision.
- Stay on the diet for seven to fourteen days, depending on
  your symptoms. Rheumatoid arthritics, for example, would
  need to stay on the diet for fourteen days (and sometimes
  longer). They would also avoid meat.
- If it's not on the list, you can't have it! As you see, no bread,
  no cake, no sauces, no cereals, no ice cream, no milk, etc.
- You can eat any amount of allowed foods, in any combination, at any time.
- You will be bored, but don't go hungry.
- You need starch for energy — eat the sweet potato at least
  three times per day.
- You should buy everything fresh. You can freeze it at home if
  you wish, because you won't add chemicals in the process.
- No smoking, no tea, no coffee.
- If you use salt, it should be pure sea salt without added
  chemicals.
- Use one to two teaspoons of Epsom salts for the first two
  days, especially if you are constipated, but not if you already
  have diarrhoea.
- Brush your teeth in bicarbonate of soda and water — toothpaste contains chemicals and corn. Put one teaspoon of bicarbonate into a glass of water, stir with your toothbrush and
  clean your teeth.
- Do not lick stamps or envelopes — the glue contains corn-
  starch and other foods.
- Check your medicines! Many drugs are packed in the factory
  with corn, potato, wheat, sugar, etc. Avoid them if you can,
  but do not stop taking a drug prescribed by your doctor without consulting first. **It is dangerous to stop medication
  without advice.**

- This is a diagnostic diet. It is therefore very important to stick *rigidly* to the allowed foods. This is *the only way* to find out if foods are causing your symptoms, or not.
- You may feel worse in the first few days with headache, muscle pain, fatigue and low mood. These are withdrawal symptoms. They feel like the flu. If they are severe, take soluble paracetamol and a hot drink of bicarbonate of soda (two teaspoons in hot water).
- It would be wise, while you're at it, to stay away from chemical exposures during this time. Remove all sources of chemical, namely anything that smells — bleach, pot-pourri, polish, perfumes, smelly soaps, etc.

Dietary investigation for food intolerance, stage 2

The Low Allergy Diet will get rid of the symptoms of food intolerance. The very fact that symptoms disappear when you stop eating your regular foods is an indication that they were caused by those foods in the first place. Conversely, whatever symptoms you have left at the end of the Low Allergy Diet cannot be blamed on the foods you haven't been eating. Therefore, if symptoms persist, abandon the investigation and seek expert help. The possibilities are:

1. You are not suffering from food intolerance, and your symptoms are due to something else entirely.
2. You are very unlucky to be intolerant to something allowed on the stage 1 diet.
3. Your symptoms are compounded by chemical sensitivity or gut fermentation.

You should proceed to stage 2 only if you have enjoyed a substantial reduction in symptoms. You are now in a position to test foods individually. The wash-out period of stage 1 accomplishes two things. Firstly, of course, it gets rid of your symptoms. Secondly, and just as important, it primes your system to react quickly to new foods as they are introduced. In other words, your intolerant reactions to food will be much more obvious now because your system has had a good wash-out. Any departure from this state of relief must be considered a reaction until proven otherwise.

In stage 2 (and 3 and 4), we will try to bring your symptoms back! We will reintroduce foods one by one, and we will identify your culprit foods in the process. Most reactions to the foods on the list below will occur within five hours of ingestion, although some foods — such as the meats — may take a little longer. Longer-reacting foods are tested in the evenings. This gives them the evening and the whole night to react (if they're going to). Thus, if you wake in the morning with a symptom, blame the new food from the night before. The golden rules are:

1. New foods should be tested *one at a time*.
2. Allow a five-hour interval between each new food.
3. Eat any safe food with the new food, or in between new foods.
4. Any symptom experienced during testing must be blamed on the last new food introduced.
5. Watch out for headache, joint pains, wheeze, runny nose, itchy skin, depression, fatigue, diarrhoea, bloating, nausea, etc., and always blame the food — don't rationalise!
6. If in doubt about a food — leave it out. It doesn't matter if a food is wrongly blamed because it can be easily retested (after a five-day gap). It does matter if you unwittingly allow a culprit food to sneak back into your diet.
7. If you get no reaction to a food consider it safe, and eat it as often as you like thereafter.
8. If you do get a reaction *stop testing new foods*! And don't eat any more new foods until you are feeling well again. Continue to eat all of your safe foods whilst you wait for the reaction to subside.
9. If the reaction is severe take soluble paracetamol and a hot drink of bicarbonate of soda (two teaspoons in water).
10. Reintroduce foods as follows:

Day	Breakfast	Lunch	Evening meal
1	Celery	Banana	Rice
2	Tomato	Carrots	Onion
3	Melon	Cauliflower	Beef
4	Tap water	Lettuce	Chicken
5	Oranges	Mushroom	Soy bean*
6	Cow's milk, one glass	Cabbage	Turkey
7	Tea — one cup only	Apple	Yeast†
8	Butter	Pineapple	Pork
9	Eggs	No new food‡	Potato
10	Cheddar cheese	No new food‡	Spinach

*Soak the beans for eight hours, boil for ninety minutes, mash into minced beef and chopped onion (if safe) and make a burger.
†Crush three tablets of yeast into a safe food.
‡Eggs and cheese may take longer than five hours to react.

Keep a detailed diary of foods eaten and symptoms experienced throughout the entire investigation:

New food tested	Time eaten	Symptoms, if any	List of safe foods
E.g. celery	Monday 8 a.m.	None	Celery
E.g. banana	Monday 1 p.m.	Headache after thirty minutes, lasted for two hours	—
E.g. rice	Monday 6 p.m	None	Rice

Dietary investigation for food intolerance, stage 3

We now move on to cereals and sugars. These are different from stage 2 foods, in that they do not always produce such an immediate reaction. They may take two or three days to produce symptoms. Thus, you could have wheat on Monday, Tuesday and Wednesday, and wake up on Thursday with a migraine. For this reason different rules apply, particularly in relation to the duration of each test. For the sake of variety, other foods are included here which will react within eight hours of ingestion.

Day	New food	Notes
1		Test in the form of wholemeal pasta, pure shredded wheat and/or home-made wholemeal bread.(use
2	Wheat	wholemeal flour — no white flour added, bread soda, an egg — if
3		safe — and buttermilk — if milk is safe). Some form of wheat must be eaten at each meal for the three full days.
4	Coffee	Freshly ground, one cup only for breakfast.
	Pepper	Black peppercorn ground on evening meal.
5	Cane sugar	Demerara or muscovado (the brown one!). Take two teaspoons at each meal for one full day.

6	Coconut	Use desiccated or creamed, with breakfast.
	Peanuts	Use the raw ground ('monkey') nut, with the evening meal.
7	Beet sugar	Standard white table sugar. Take two teaspoons at each meal for one full day.
8 9	Corn	Use in two forms: corn on the cob and glucose powder. Also use home-made popcorn and pure cornflour if you like. Start each meal with fresh corn on the cob, and finish with two teaspoons of glucose powder.
10	Cauliflower Garlic	For breakfast. With the evening meal.
11 12	Oats	Test in the form of porridge, oatcakes and/or flapjacks (oat flake, safe sugar, butter). Eat some form of oat at each meal for two full days.
13	Malt	Use the extract, mix two teaspoons into a safe food at each meal for the full day.
14 15	Rye	Test in the form of Ryvita crispbread or pure rye bread. Eat some at each meal for two full days.

NB: Remember, if you wake up in the morning with symptoms blame the last new food from the day before. Abandon a test as soon as you are sure that a reaction has occurred.

Dietary investigation for food intolerance, stage 4

You now know which staple foods are safe and which ones cause you trouble. We now move on to stage 4. This is an open-ended stage, and it can go on as long as you like. During the first seven days we pay special attention to some of the chemicals added to food by man. Thereafter we test foods with multiple ingredients.

Day	New food	Notes
1	White bread	(Test only if wheat is safe!) This is a test for anti-caking agents, bleaching agents, etc.
2	Frozen peas	These are treated with sulphur dioxide and other chemicals.
3	Instant coffee	This is roasted over an ethylene gas flame and contains many chemicals.
4	Tinned carrots	If you are safe with fresh carrots, but react to tinned carrots in water (phenolic resin lining the can), you will have to be careful with all tinned foods.
5	Monosodium glutamate	This is used as a flavour enhancer, especially in Chinese food.
6	Saccharin	This is a sweetener hidden in some soft drinks and confectionery. Take two tablets as a test.
7	Raisins	These are also treated with sulphur dioxide.

You can now proceed to foods with multiple ingredients. This includes jams, sauces, chocolate, cake, biscuits, etc. However, don't forget all of the other possibilities: cucumber, grapefruit, dates, asparagus, lemon, lentils, prawns, sprouts, chickpea, almonds, herring, sunflower seeds, etc. If you get a reaction from a food with multiple ingredients, you should be able to trace the source of your trouble (because you know your status with the main ingredients).

Dietary investigation for food intolerance: troubleshooting

This is for patients who enjoy great relief from symptoms on the Low Allergy Diet, and then get confused. Their symptoms may have recurred without clear-cut reactions. In the first place, let me say this: never lose sight of the fact that you have food intolerance! Get expert help if you cannot figure out your culprit foods. There are several sources of confusion:

1. *You have allowed a culprit food to sneak into your diet.* Go back to the point where you last felt well and eat only those foods which you are sure of. Stay there for a few days until

symptoms clear again. Retest the foods, but this time *take larger portions.*

2. *Your reactions take longer than five hours.* Go back to the point where you last felt well and eat only those foods which you are sure of. Stay there for a few days until symptoms clear again. Retest the foods, but this time give them longer to react. For example, allow one full day per stage 2 food; test wheat over one full week, etc.

3. *You have gut fermentation.* In this case symptoms will slowly return with a build-up of carbohydrate (starch and sugar) foods. Have a gut fermentation test (see below).

4. *You're drinking too much caffeine.* You had no reaction to one cup of tea (or coffee), you correctly thought you were not intolerant, and you started to drink too much of it. Stick to one cup of tea and one cup of coffee per day until the investigation is complete. Increase your consumption thereafter if you wish.

5. *Chemicals are accumulating.* Symptoms may result from the accumulation of natural and/or added chemicals as you expand your diet.

Dietary investigation complete! Now what?

You have now completed your dietary investigation for food intolerance. You have two options:

1. You can avoid your culprit foods. You may find that you can tolerate small amounts of your culprit foods after a prolonged period of abstinence, say six to twelve months. See what you can get away with!

2. You can opt for a course of Enzyme Potentiated Desensitisation (see chapter 18). This will increase your tolerance to culprit foods, and allow you to eat them without the penalty of illness. If you have had multiple reactions, or if your culprit foods are hard to avoid socially and nutritionally, you should give this treatment serious consideration.

Meanwhile . . .

- Try to vary the diet as much as possible. This will help to prevent the development of new 'allergies'.
- Regular vigorous exercise is beneficial to the body in general, and to the immune system in particular.
- Beware of food cravings, they signal the emergence of new intolerance.

5. The chemical holiday

Patients who suspect they have chemical sensitivity should organise a chemical 'holiday', i.e. a fortnight away from chemicals. This involves considerable upheaval in our modern world. The aim of the 'holiday' is to see whether symptoms disappear or not. If they do, chemical sensitivity is a real possibility; if they don't, it's not. The ideal holiday involves admission to an Environmental Control Unit. This is a highly specialised hospital unit which ensures a chemical-free environment. All of the materials used in the construction of the unit are chemical-free, and all of the air is filtered to prevent the entry of pollutants. The unit is kept under positive pressure, which means that there is a draught from the inside out, rather than the converse. Staff and visitors are careful not to bring chemicals into the unit by means of freshly polished footwear, dry-cleaned clothes, perfume, aftershave, hair gel, and so on. Visitors who appear with chemical smells are offered a shower and a change of clothes before they are allowed in. If they refuse, they are politely asked to return another day more suitably prepared! Symptoms of chemical sensitivity quickly disappear in such a unit. Patients are then tested in a special booth for their sensitivity to individual chemicals. (This is part of the research being carried out on veterans with Gulf War Syndrome.)

However, such units are expensive and are reserved for those who can afford it, and those who really need it. In practice, most chemically sensitive patients get away with arranging their own chemical holiday. The first requirement is a house not polluted by petrochemical heating fumes: in other words, a house free of gas, oil, kerosene, etc. An all-electric house is ideal, or one where the heating boiler is in a separate shed. Stay with a co-operative friend if you need to — we did!* Rid the house of everything that smells. You will need to recruit the co-operation of all household members to achieve this. Do not use cosmetics, air fresheners, polish, etc. Keep all windows and doors open to ventilate the house, weather permitting. If all symptoms disappear, return home and follow the instructions for the chemically sensitive. These measures will increase your tolerance to small amounts of chemical. If you find that symptoms are still too easily provoked, consider a course of Enzyme Potentiated Desensitisation. This will increase your tolerance further.

---

*Aoife's story is covered in *Feeling Tired All the Time*.

6. Tests for 'candida' and gut fermentation

If the skin-prick test is negative, you are not allergic to candida! Gut fermentation is a completely different condition and can be easily confirmed by a positive fermentation test. The test procedure is simple, but it needs to be interpreted by a doctor with an interest:

1. No alcohol for twenty-four hours before the test.
2. Observe a total fast for three hours before the test.
3. Take one gram of glucose in capsule form with four grams of glucose diluted in water.
4. One hour later, whilst you are still fasting, a blood sample is drawn, and sent to Biolab, London. (For address, see appendix 2.)
5. It measures the blood levels of various alcohols: ethanol, methanol, propanol and butanol.
6. Fermentation is confirmed by elevated levels.
7. The source of fermentation (bacterial or yeast) is known by the type of alcohol produced.

7. The Good, the Bad and the Ugly

There is seldom a perfectly reliable test in medicine, and all of the tests listed above have varying degrees of sensitivity and specificity. They are good but they are not perfect, and they are not an end in themselves. They must always be interpreted in the context of the whole of things. This is true of all medical tests, but never more so than in the case of allergy. The dietary and chemical tests, in particular, are subjective. They depend on a patient's experience of symptom relief and recurrence. They are, therefore, at the mercy of the placebo effect, and all of the other variables of human nature. In spite of this obvious drawback, many patients find lasting relief from their symptoms by using these methods.

We cannot leave this topic without reference to the plethora of 'alternative allergy tests' on offer: vega testing, radionics, pendulum swinging, divination, kinesiology, pulse testing, etc. These all claim the ability to tell you, in a jiffy, what you're allergic to. A few blood tests also lay claim to the same magical ability. The latter are more ominous than the former because they have a semblance of science about them, but it's nothing more than pseudo-science. There is no rational basis for any of these tests; they are neither sensitive nor specific, and they give rise to endless false positives and negatives. In short, they are useless. Their attraction, from the patient's point of view, is that they offer a quick and easy solution, and they preclude the need for painstaking dietary investigation.

Many food-intolerant patients have been told by orthodox medicine that they are 'not allergic' when they know well they are. Thus dismissed, they seek out a practitioner who will respect their intelligence! Perhaps you are one of these? 'I had my allergies tested in this way,' you may say, 'and it worked!' Great — I have no problem with that. You stopped eating certain foods and you got better. You probably do have food intolerance, but that does not justify the diagnostic method!

Let me illustrate what I mean. Imagine we have in front of us 100 people with food intolerance, and let's suppose they are all eating a standard Western European diet. We put a dartboard on the wall, and we replace numbers on the board with the names of our staple foods. We don a blindfold and throw ten darts at the board. Then we tell *all* of our patients to avoid the following foods: wheat, yeast, sugars, dairy produce, caffeine, chocolate, and citrus fruit. We also throw in a few extras here and there on an individual basis to make it look good. Our result is guaranteed: 25 per cent will improve within fourteen days. We have just invented a new diagnostic test for allergies: it's the 'blindfold dartboard test'! We would vary it a little, of course. If we were dealing with a North American population, for example, we would advise our patients to avoid peanuts and corn; and an Asian population would avoid rice and soy bean. Why? Because, as a general rule, we become intolerant to the foods we most commonly eat. Excluding these foods will therefore lead to an improvement in food-related symptoms.

However, there are several problems with our blindfold dartboard test:

1. It's not specific enough. Our patients do not know whether one, or two, or indeed all of the omitted foods are causing their trouble. The 'diagnosis' is incomplete.
2. It's not sensitive enough. It neglects the 75 per cent who do not improve, and leads them to believe they are not food-intolerant when they are.
3. It leads to incomplete treatment. Some patients have been advised to stick to very severe regimes for years on end. They are socially inconvenienced (to say the least), and they are at risk of nutritional deficiency.

251

In conclusion, then, our new test is quite useless — in spite of the fact that it 'works' some of the time.

Please understand that I have no wish to belittle alternative or complementary medicine in all of this. On the contrary, I believe it has a lot to offer, not least in its espousal of a holistic approach to medicine. Furthermore, the genuine practitioners of alternative therapies would share the concerns I have outlined above. Besides, the pseudo-scientific useless blood tests alluded to above are promoted by practitioners of orthodox training!

18 The Effective Treatment of Allergy

The principles for the effective treatment of allergy are briefly summarised thus:

1. Identify the thing(s) you are allergic to.
2. Avoid the thing(s) you are allergic to.
3. Take medication to deal with your symptoms.
4. Desensitise.

The first two principles here are obvious, and have been dealt with at relevant points throughout the book. The third principle, the prescription of medication, is a matter for individual discussion with your own doctor. It would be quite wrong for me to offer generalisations on this issue, and for this reason, I have deliberately stayed away from naming drugs and suggesting doses. I would like to dedicate this final chapter to Dr Len McEwen, the pioneer who developed a very specific and effective treatment for allergy, namely Enzyme Potentiated Desensitisation, or EPD for short.

The story of EPD goes back to 1959, and to the London office of an ear, nose and throat surgeon named Popper. He was interested in nasal polyps, those grape-like structures that can block a nose. He knew that polyps consisted mainly of a gooey substance called hyaluronic acid, and he figured that if he could dissolve the acid, the polyp would shrink, and the patient could avoid surgery. Nice thought! He injected his patients' nasal polyps with an enzyme (hyaluronidase) which he hoped would break down the acid. When they returned for a progress report, they volunteered that their polyps were still there, *but some of them had stopped sneezing.* In other words, the injection had desensitised them. They no longer had allergic rhinitis.

Popper then tried to repeat his experiment with another batch of hyaluronidase and another batch of patients. However, this time he failed to desensitise. Sadly, his work was cut short by an untimely death. That would have been the end of the story if it were not for the ingenuity and persistence of Dr Len McEwen. He knew from Popper's work that hyaluronidase was not the important ingredient, and realised that the first batch must have been contaminated with some other active ingredient. He went back to this batch and found six contaminants. By trial and error he found the gem, an enzyme called beta-glucuronidase. He successfully desensitised both animals and man to various allergens, and his findings were published in the medical literature. He has devoted his working life to the further development of this treatment.

What is EPD?

EPD is a desensitisation treatment for allergy. It consists of a mixture of beta-glucuronidase and allergens. The enzyme is already present in our bodies and has powerful immune system effects. The allergen mixtures include commonly eaten foods, airborne allergens, chemicals and a few 'odds and ends'. Each patient will receive the allergen mixture best suited to their needs.

How does it work?

A very small amount (0.05 ml) of EPD solution is injected between two layers of skin. The enzyme stimulates special cells in the skin called antigen presenting cells (APCs). These 'wake up' to find themselves bathed in the allergen mixture. They lay hold of the allergens and migrate to the immune system 'headquarters'. Their job in life is to present allergen and ask for judgment: 'Do we ignore this allergen or do we mount an immune response against it?' Because the APCs are primed with beta-glucuronidase, the immune system responds favourably to the allergen, realises there is no threat to health, and organises a truce. A new population of cells is then called forth with instructions not to react in the presence of these allergens. These cells are called T suppressor cells. They have the power of a military police force, and they suppress other components of the immune system which would otherwise react to the allergen. T suppressor cells suppress allergic reactions.

What is it used for?

EPD has been used successfully in the treatment of hay fever, asthma, perennial rhinitis, nasal polyps, urticaria and angioedema, as well as food-induced hyperactivity, migraine, Irritable Bowel Syndrome, Crohn's disease, ulcerative colitis, eczema and arthritis. It has also helped some patients with Chronic Fatigue Syndrome. EPD has not yet been developed for the treatment of contact allergic dermatitis, drug allergy or insect sting allergy.

Is it safe?

The amount of allergen administered with each dose of EPD is never greater than the dose you would receive with a diagnostic skin-prick test. For this reason, EPD is a very safe treatment. Patients with a history of life-threatening allergic reactions are offered an even greater degree of safety: an epidermal scrape. This consists of superficially scraping the skin with the edge of a blunted scalpel. A sterile plastic 'cup' is then taped over the scrape, and filled with EPD treatment. The solution is allowed to percolate through the skin over twenty-four hours, and the cup is then removed. Some fluid may still be present, and a jelly-like substance may cover the scrape. This will dry within thirty minutes, and the scrape will heal normally over the next ten days or so. There have been no serious side effects from EPD since its inception some thirty years ago.

Are there any side effects?

It is quite normal for the injection site to swell immediately after injection. This will quickly subside. A delayed swelling may also occur after three to six hours and may persist for three days, but it should begin to subside by the fourth day. Very rarely, the whole forearm may swell. These are not serious reactions and they respond to antihistamine tablets. Other side effects include a transient worsening of the allergies being treated, such as sneezing, runny nose, urticaria, etc. These will usually disappear within a few days, but may persist in some cases for a few weeks, and very rarely, for a few months. Patients undergoing a course of EPD are given detailed instructions. This will increase their chance of success and keep side effects to a minimum.

Is it effective?

EPD has been shown by clinical trial to be effective in up to 80 per cent of patients. In other words, four out of five patients whose allergies have been properly identified will enjoy some benefit from treatment.

How long will it be before improvement?

It takes about twenty-one days for the newly stimulated T-cells to mature. There will usually be no appreciable difference in your allergic symptoms until this time has elapsed. The response to the first dose of EPD is variable — most patients will experience some benefit, but some may not, and some may even feel worse. Patients with eczema, hyperactivity and Chronic Fatigue Syndrome are most likely to report a definite, albeit transient, worsening of symptoms after their first dose of EPD. Subsequent doses do not have a negative effect.

How many injections will I need?

Simple allergies such as house dust mite will respond to two or three injections. Significant relief from hay fever may be obtained by just one or two injections given well before your hay fever season starts. Other conditions may require four injections (or more) before any real improvement is noticed. Injections are given at intervals of eight to twelve weeks until a good response is obtained. Then, depending on response, the injections are given at ever-increasing intervals. Once their symptoms are well controlled, most patients find that they can stop injections for very long periods. Relapses may occur after five or six years and these respond to booster doses.

EPD, not to be confused with Blocking Desensitisation (Incremental Immunotherapy)

Blocking desensitisation is a technique which involves injections of allergen in incremental doses. The first injection is small, the second is a little stronger than the first, the third a little stronger than the second, and so forth. This method of desensitisation floods the immune system with allergen, and provokes the production of a 'blocking antibody'. This is an immunoglobulin which saturates the mast cells and basophils, and in so doing prevents their degranulation by IgE. The system was developed in the late nineteenth century. It works well, and is still used today throughout continental Europe and North America. However, it has caused a number of deaths from anaphylaxis — just like the unfortunate dogs of Richet and Portier (see chapter 9). For this very good reason, blocking desensitisation is not used at all in Ireland, and is used only in highly specialised centres in the United Kingdom. The technique is limited to specific allergens, such as grass pollen, insect venom and house dust mite. Incremental immunotherapy is the only effective desensitisation technique for insect venom anaphylaxis.

EPD uses much smaller doses than blocking desensitisation, and for this reason is a much safer technique. It also has a wider scope in that it can be used for many allergens simultaneously.

Where can I get more information on EPD?

Check out the Website: http://www.epdallergy.com/epd/epdhome.

Check out the British Society for Allergy, Environmental and Nutritional Medicine (see appendix 2).

Appendix 1
A Word about
House Dust Mites

It's official: the World Health Organization has formally declared that the humble house dust mite is a universal health problem! It causes trouble for patients with asthma, rhinitis and eczema. The mite is a tiny relative of spiders and ticks. It lives in bedding, carpets, upholstery, teddy bears, and the like. It lives off the skin flakes we shed, and shed them we do. It prefers a temperature range between 22 and 26°C, and a relative humidity greater than 55 per cent. Thus, the tight buildings we have developed in the Western world greatly favour the mite. Wall-to-wall carpets, central heating, double-glazed windows and luxurious bedding all provide the domestic mite with an ideal environment in which to thrive. Actually, it's not the mites themselves that cause trouble; it's the droppings they leave behind. Specifically, it's the digestive enzymes on the faecal pellets which cause the allergy. There may be several pounds' weight of dust mite faeces in a single mattress! These pellets are microscopic and easily become airborne. Vacuum cleaning, for example, throws the allergen into the air, and leaves it suspended there for several hours. Reducing your exposure to the mite allergen will result in a reduction of symptoms. In fact, asthma symptoms may be reduced by up to 50 per cent in this way. Eczema and rhinitis will also improve. Obviously, there is no point in going to the expense of avoidance measures if you are not allergic to the mite, so get a skin test before adopting the following:

- Concentrate on the bedroom, you spend a third of your life there!
- Sleep with the window open, or consider the use of an air filter.

- Use an allergen exclusion bedding system, such as Alprotec.*
This will prevent the dust mite from travelling in and out of
your mattress, duvet and pillow.
- Air the bedding well each day.
- Wash bedding at over 55°C. This kills the mite.
- Use a denaturing anti-dust mite spray (from your pharmacy).
- Use smooth flooring, such as linoleum, cork or wood. Carpets
are a rich source of dust mites, and they are hard to clean. A
smooth floor can be damp-dusted.
- Damp-dust regularly; do not use dry dusters.
- Light curtains are preferred, they are easier to wash and
should be washed at regular intervals.
- Minimum amounts of books, knick-knacks and plants. They
are dust (and mould) traps.
- Use a vacuum cleaner which has a special filter, or fit a filter
to your existing cleaner if you can. The filter should state
'blocks 99.95% of particles greater than 0.3 microns'. This will
allow you to vacuum without fear of throwing too much
allergen into the air.
- Teddy bear care (and other soft toys): freeze overnight and
wash on a weekly basis.

---

*Advanced Allergy Technologies Ltd, Freepost ALM1541, Altrincham, Cheshire, WA15 0BR.

Appendix 2
Useful Addresses

Action against Allergy
24–6 High Street
Hampton Hill
Middlesex TW12 1PD
England
Offers information, mail order books, films and lectures on allergy and related topics.

Anaphylaxis Campaign (Ireland)
PO Box 4373
Dublin 18
Ireland
Tel: (01) 2952791

Anaphylaxis Campaign (UK)
PO Box 149
Fleet
Hants. GU13 9XU
England
Tel: (01252) 318723

Asthma Society of Ireland
Eden House
15–17 Eden Quay
Dublin 1
Ireland
Tel: (01) 8788511

Biolab Medical Unit
The Stone House
9 Weymouth Street
London W1N 3FF
England
Tel: (0171) 6365959
A specialised unit which provides laboratory assessment of nutritional status, and expert advice (by consultation).

British Association for Counselling
1 Regent Place
Rugby
Warwickshire CV21 2PJ
England

British Society for Allergy and Clinical Immunology
66 Weston Park
Thames Ditton
Surrey KT7 0HL
England
Tel: (0181) 3982766
Provides a list of Allergy Clinics available on the National Health Service to which you may be referred by your doctor.

British Society for Allergy, Environmental and Nutritional Medicine (BSAENM)
PO Box 28
Totton
Southampton SO40 2ZA
England
Tel: (01703) 812124
A society of doctors with a special interest in allergy and related issues. Will provide your doctor with a list of medical practitioners to whom you may be referred.

Hyperactive Children's Support Group
71 Whyke Lane
Chichester
East Sussex PO19 2LD
England
Tel: (01903) 725182

Irish ME Trust
18 Upper Fitzwilliam Street
Dublin 2
Ireland
Tel: (01) 6761413

ME Association (UK)
Stanhope House
High Street
Stanford-le-Hope
Essex SS17 OAH
England
Tel: (01375) 642466
An organisation which provides support and information for patients with ME. Information on support groups in your area is available.

Medic Alert
12 Bridge Wharf
156 Caledonian Road
London N1 9UU
England
Tel: (0171) 8333034
For registering serious allergy problems (and other medical disorders).

National Eczema Society
163 Eversholt Street
London NW1 1BU
England
Tel: (0171) 3884800

Pesticide Exposure Group of Sufferers
3 Lloyds House
Regent Terrace
Cambridge CB2 1AA
England
Tel: (01223) 64707

Psychological Society of Ireland
13 Adelaide Road
Dublin 2
Ireland
Tel: (01) 4783916

Appendix 3
Bibliography

Feeling Tired All the Time
Dr Joe Fitzgibbon
Dublin: Gill & Macmillan, 1993
ISBN 0 7171 2101 1

The Complete Guide to Food Allergy and Intolerance
Dr Jonathon Brostoff and Linda Gamlin
London: Bloomsbury, 1989
ISBN 0 7475 0242 0

The Migraine Revolution
J. Mansfield
Northamptonshire: Thorsons, 1986
ISBN 0 7225 1314 3

Arthritis: Allergy, Nutrition and the Environment
J. Mansfield
Northamptonshire: Thorsons, 1995
ISBN 07225 1903 6

And for the scientifically minded:

Environmental Medicine in Clinical Practice
H. Anthony, S. Birtwistle, K. Eaton and J. Maberly
Southampton: BSAENM Publications, 1997 (for address see
appendix 2)
ISBN 0 9523397 2 2

Food Allergy and Intolerance
Dr Jonathon Brostoff and S.J. Challacombe (eds.)
London: Balliere Tindall, London, 1987
ISBN 0 7020 1156 8

Allergy and Allergic Diseases, 2 vols.
A.B. Kay (ed.)
Oxford: Blackwell Science Ltd, Osney Mead, 1997
ISBN 0 86542 867 0

Allergic Diseases: Diagnosis and Management, 4th edn
R. Patterson, L. Grammer, P.A. Greenberger and C.R. Zeiss
Philadelphia: J.B. Lipincott Company, 1993
ISBN 0 397 51126 4

Food Allergy: Adverse Reactions to Foods and Food Additives
D. Metcalfe, H.A. Sampson and R.A. Simon (eds.)
Oxford: Blackwell Scientific Publications, 1991
ISBN 0 86542 094 7

Allergy: Theory and Practice, 2nd edn
P.E. Korenblat and H.J. Wedner (eds.)
Philadelphia: W.B. Saunders Company, 1992
ISBN 0 7216 7244 4

Food and Food Additive Intolerance in Children
T.J. David
Oxford: Blackwell Scientific Publications, 1993
ISBN 0 632 03487 4

Principles and Practice of Immunotoxicology
K. Miller, J. Turk and S. Nicklin
Oxford: Blackwell Scientific Publications, 1992
ISBN 0 632 02563 8

Diets for Sick Children, 4th edn
D. Francis
Oxford: Blackwell Scientific Publications, 1987
ISBN 0 632 00505 X

Lecture Notes on Occupational Medicine, 4th edn
H.A. Waldron
Oxford: Blackwell Scientific Publications, 1990
ISBN 0 632 02764 9

Fisher's Contact Dermatitis, 4th edn
R.L. Rietschel and J.F. Fowler, Jr
Baltimore: Williams and Wilkins, 1995
ISBN 0 683 07282 X

Dermatology, 3rd edn, 2 vols.
S.L. Moschella and H.J. Hurley (eds.)
Philadelphia: W.B. Saunders Company, 1992
ISBN 0 7216 3263 7

Handbook of Clinical Allergy
N.C. Thomson, E.M. Kirkwood and R.S. Lever
Oxford: Blackwell Scientific Publications, 1990
ISBN 0 632 02676 6

Stress, the Immune System and Psychiatry
B.E. Leonard and K. Miller (eds.)
Chichester: Wiley, 1995
ISBN 0 471 95258 3

Post-Viral Fatigue Syndrome
Drs R. Jenkins and J.F. Mowbray (eds.)
Chichester: Wiley, 1991
ISBN 0 471 92846 1

Postviral Fatigue Syndrome
P.O. Behan, D.P. Goldberg and J.F. Mowbray (eds.)
British Medical Bulletin, vol. 47, no. 4, October 1991
Churchill Livingston
ISBN 0 443 044902

Clinical Management of Chronic Fatigue Syndrome
N. Klimas and R. Patarca (eds.)
New York: The Haworth Medical Press, 1995
ISBN 1 56024 792 4

The Clinical and Scientific Basis of ME/CFS
B.M. Hyde
Ottawa: The Nightingale Research Foundation, 1992
ISBN 0 9695662 0 4

Index